Malaria Research in Southeast Asia

MALARIA RESEARCH IN SOUTHEAST ASIA

VIROJ WIWANITKIT

Nova Science Publishers, Inc.
New York

LIBRARY OF CONGRESS CATALOGING-IN-PUBLICATION DATA

Viroj Wiwanitkit.
Malaria research in Southeast Asia / Viroj Wiwanitkit.
p. ; cm.
Includes bibliographical references and index.
ISBN-13: 978-1-60021-821-7 (hardcover)
ISBN-10: 1-60021-821-0 (hardcover)
1. Malaria--Southeast Asia. 2. Malaria--Research--Southeast Asia. I. Title.
[DNLM: 1. Malaria--Asia, Southeastern. 2. Arthropod Vectors--Asia, Southeastern. WC 750 V819m 2007]
RC164.S64V56 2007
616.9'36200959--dc22
2007025118

Published by Nova Science Publishers, Inc. ✢ New York

CONTENTS

Chapter 1

Introduction to Mosquito-Borne Disease

Abstract

Infection is still an important problem in the present day. Vector-borne disease is an important group of infectious diseases. A vector-borne disease is a disease in which the pathogenic microorganism is transmitted from an infected individual to another individual by an arthropod or other agent, sometimes with other animals serving as intermediary hosts. In this article, introduction to mosquito-borne diseases can be found.

Mosquito-Borne Diseases, an Important Member of Vector-Borne Diseases

Infection is still an important problem in the present day. Vector-borne disease is an important group of infectious diseases. A vector-borne disease is a disease in which the pathogenic microorganism is transmitted from an infected individual to another individual by an arthropod or other agent, sometimes with other animals serving as intermediary hosts [1]. The transmission depends upon the attributes and requirements of at least three different living organisms: the pathologic agent, either virus, protozoa, parasite or bacteria; the vector, which are commonly arthropods such as ticks or mosquitoes; and the human host [1 - 2] (Figure 1). In addition, intermediary hosts such as domesticated and/or wild animals often serve as a reservoir for the pathogen until susceptible human populations are exposed [1 - 2].

Of several arthropod-related vector-borne disease, mosquito-borne diseases are worldwide mentioned. Mosquito is considered as a dangerous animal in the world, killing millions people per year. In Southeast Asian, there is an ancient verbal that "mosquito is more dangerous than tiger." In medicine, Mosquitoes can carry many different kinds of diseases including malaria, filariasis, dirofilariasis, dengue fever, encephalitis and yellow fever (Table 1). Therefore, the mosquito-borne disease is still an important infectious disease at present. Due to the globalization in the present day, the change in the epidemiology of diseases from one site to the others all around the world can be expected. The summative on the common mosquito-borne diseases in the tropical countries can be and should be performed. That work can be a useful reference material for the practitioners who are not familiar to the unique problems of the developing world and might face up with those problems due to the possible migration of diseases. Schlagenhauf noted that an estimated 50 to 70 million Western travelers are exposed to malaria infection annually [3]. Green and Roberts recently said that the threat to the package tourist differed greatly from that to the businessman, soldier or backpacker [4]. They noted that latter groups may have little control over their food and water supplies and be exposed to vector-borne and zoonotic infections normally restricted to remote locations [4]. They also noted that the common factor was that all such infections might be transported around the world within their incubation period, and that any disease can now present to any doctor [4]. They concluded that today more than ever before it was incumbent on any practitioner to ask not only 'where have you been?' but also 'what were you doing there?' [4].

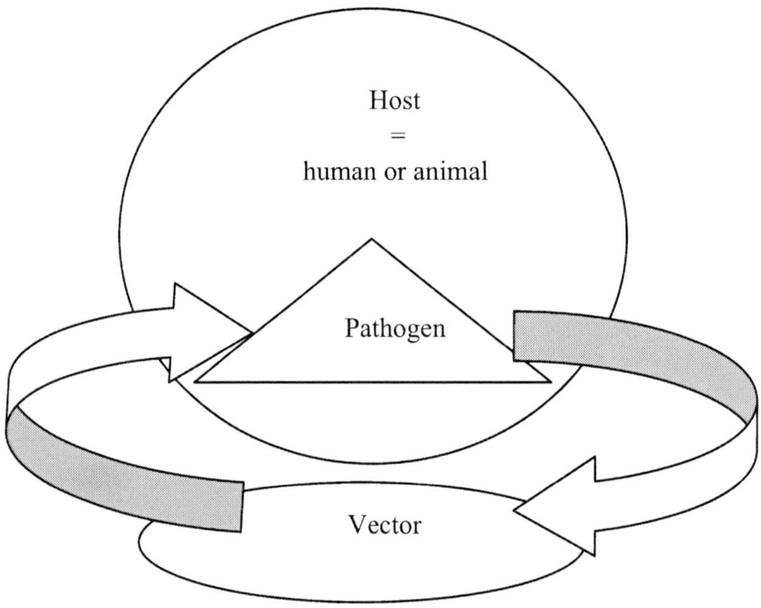

Figure 1 The composition of a vector-borne diseases

Table 1 Examples of some important vector-borne diseases [1 – 2]

Groups	Examples
Mosquito-borne disease	Malaria, filariasis, dengue fever, yellow fever
Tick-borne disease	Ehrlichiosis, babesiosis, anaplasmosis, Q fever
Flea-borne disease	Murine typhus
Lice-borne disease	Trench fever
Fly-borne disease	Turalemia, sleeping sickness
Lice-borne disease	Rickettsial pox

EXAMPLE OF IMPORTANT MOSQUITO-BORNE DISEASES

As previously mentioned, there are several infectious diseases in the mosquito-borne diseases group. These diseases can be seen all over the world. Some of medically important mosquito-borne diseases are

A. Malaria

Malaria is a protozoan infection transmitted by the biting female Anopheles mosquito. These mosquitoes bite during the nighttime hours, from dusk to dawn. It cannot be casually transmitted from person to person but it is possible to spread malaria via blood or placenta transfusions [1 – 2]. Symptoms of malaria include fever, shivering, pain and vomiting [5]. Some serious presentation such as generalized convulsions and coma are also documented [1 – 2]. However, some uncommon presentation of malarial infection such as epistaxis and hypermenorrhea are mentioned [5]. In addition, as many as half a billion people worldwide are left with chronic anemia due to malaria infections. The malarial symptoms of the disease usually begin 1 week to 2 weeks after being bit [1 – 2].

According to the World Health Organization, malaria infects between 300 and 500 million people every year in Africa, South Asia, Southeast Asia, the Middle East, Oceania, and Central and South America. The disease affects approximately 40% of the world's population and over one million of the infected die each year [3]. The corresponding pathogen is *Plasmodium* spp. It is the most well known mosquito-borne disease. For several centuries, this disease has been documented as an important threatens to humans. In addition, it is important problem for farm animals especially chicken. There is also a specific museum for malaria. In the Museum for the History of the Pavia University, Italy, important materials on the role of this scientist in the history of malariology are kept [6]. Malaria is accepted as one of the most important tropical infectious disease. However, the spread of malaria to the non-tropical countries has been mentioned for years.

Reiter noted that present global temperature was in a warming phase, which begun 200 to 300 years before [7]. Reiter noted that the potential effects of the weather included predictions that malaria would emerge from the tropics and become established in Europe and North America [7]. Until the second half of the 20th century, malaria was endemic and widespread in many temperate regions, with major epidemics as far north as the Arctic Circle [7]. From 1564 to the 1730s the coldest period of the Little Ice Age malaria was an important cause of illness and death in several parts of England [7]. Transmission began to decline only in the 19th century, when the present warming trend was well under way [7 - 8]. In Italy, there are many roman Archivio Storico Capitolino papers reconstructing the history of malaria in the city of Rome and in the countryside from 1870 to the 2nd post-war period [9]. The papers of the VIII Bureau of Hygiene and Sanity offered interesting points of views for the period 1883-1940, useful for deeply investigating the attitude of Roman Administration towards the fight against malaria [9]. Malaria is also important infection for many other European countries [10]. There are also about thousands of malaria cases reported each year in the USA, mostly by people who were infected abroad. The importance of malaria for non-tropical countries is therefore emerged. Malaria should be included in the differential diagnosis in the cases with unknown origin of fever in the traveler who had the history of visit to the endemic area [11].

Julvez noted that parasites and their vectors have been imported in many cases of insular malaria in the southwestern Indian Ocean [12]. Schlagenhauf said that malaria owed its distribution worldwide to human travelers, and travelers are linked with the discovery, refinement, and development of several antimalarial drugs [3]. It is noted that traveling to a tropical country where Malaria is present, antimalarial drug should be taken at least two weeks prior to leaving to prevent malaria [13]. It should also be noted that malaria has become resistant to the most frequently used antibiotics in some parts of the world [13]. Schlagenhauf also noted that the genomes for humans, mosquito, and Plasmodium have been completed at present, but no malaria vaccine is available as yet [3]. Control of malaria is important topic in public health. Najera noted that searching for realistic approaches to malaria control, led to the adoption of the global malaria control strategy in Amsterdam in 1992, and the challenge, at the end of the century, to rally forces commensurate with the magnitude of the problem, while aiming at realistic objectives [13]. However, there are many conflicting views on the relations between malaria and socio-economic development and the desirable integration of malaria control into sustainable development [13].

B. Filariasis and Drofilariasis

Filaria worm, a parasite in Superfamily Filariodea is an important blood parasite. Lymphatic filariasis, caused by filarial nematode parasites, is an important mosquito-borne disease in the tropical countries. Human lymphatic filariasis is a major tropical disease in which clinical manifestations range from asymptomatic microfilaraemia to chronic pathology [14 - 15]. Up to billion of people around the world is the population at risk for filariasis [16]. Hoerauf noted that infections with the filarial nematodes affect more than 150 million people mainly in the tropics [17]. The endemic area for this disease is the tropical zone, as previously mentioned, in many developing with low socioeconomic conditions. The main pathology of filariais is lymphatic filariasis, resulted from a complex interplay of the pathogenic potential of the parasite and the immune response of the host [18]. The disability due to lymphatic filariasis is of concern.

The traditional method of diagnosing filarial infections is to examine blood or skin samples for microfilariae and for many reasons, this is still the standard procedure [19]. Although the widely used screening technique at present is the microscopy technique, which is not as sensitive as the immunology or molecular technique, high prevalence of filariasis can be detected. Since the present global campaign to eliminate lymphatic filariasis new diagnostic tools have emerged like PCR, antigen detection using finger-prick blood taken during the day and ultrasound to visualize adult worm [19]. Walther and Muller recently said that the last two tests could be applied in endemic countries with limited resources and enable the detection of early infections and both tests were also particularly important for the individual in control schemes since recent researches had shown that damage was usually caused long before symptoms appeared [19]. However, the microscopy technique is still recommended in the tropical developing countries, the endemic area, due to the limitation of resource in those countries [20]. If no strict control by effective screening, filariais may re-emerge as a big problem in those communities [21].

In addition to the present strategies, which focus early detection of the microfilaria among the local population in the endemic area, the screening program should be implemented for not only the endemic area but also the non-endemic area with high density of migrant workers [20, 22 - 23]. Furthermore, effective vector control should also be concerned. Sensitive, specific, practical and acceptable screening technique for the field surveillance must be set.

Hoerauf noted that the very successful efforts to control filarial infections, however, had to be sustained by new tools that require long-term commitment to research [17]. Hoerauf said that dramatic improvement had been achieved in the control of lymphatic filariasis and onchocerciasis by vector control and mass treatment with microfilaricidal drugs [17]. Hoerauf also said that additional tools that could help in regional elimination or, ultimately, eradication of filariasis might arise from the development of new drugs or a vaccine [17]. Ivermectin, a parasiticide that long ago proved its worth in veterinary medicine, became one of the most effective tools for control programs against human filarial diseases in the 1980s [24]. Richard-Lenoble *et al* said that this drug was provided at no cost, was effective against microfilariae (blocking their transmission) and could be administered annually as a single oral dose with virtually no side-effects [24]. Richard-Lenoble *et al* also noted that these considerations led the WHO to officially declared eradicable two endemic filarial diseases (among the major endemic diseases worldwide), onchocerciasis and lymphatic filariasis [24]. Recently, Hoerauf proposed that research into the immune responses mediating protection or pathology had provided new insights into the pathways that lead to effector function and immunosuppression, such as T regulatory responses, as well as into genetic predispositions from the host's side, and to the identification of vaccine candidates that show protection in animal models [17]. Hoerauf noted that recognition of the role the Wolbachia endosymbionts might play in activating the innate immune system has altered our understanding of immunopathology of filariasis and adverse reactions to microfilaricidal drugs. Conclusively, *Wolbachia* spp. have also proven to be a new suitable targets for the development of a long-term sterilizing or potentially macrofilaricidal drug [25].

In addition to the human filaria, the dog parasites *Dirofilaria immitis and D. repens* can also occur in humans but do not produce microfilariae in them [19]. These parasites are documented as causative agents for tropical diseases in many countries. Walther and Muller noted that ELISAs and PCR probes had been devised and can usefully differentiate between pulmonary dirofilariasis and lung cancer [19]. Concern for the dirofilariasis as emerging infectious diseases is important at present.

C. Dengue Fever

Dengue virus is an arthropod-borne viral agent. There are four dengue virus serotypes: DEN-1, DEN-2, DEN-3, and DEN-4. All can cause dengue infection. Dengue infection is a major public health problem, yearly affecting numerous of children in the tropical region [26]. Dengue fever is found in infected Aedes mosquitoes and cannot be directly transmitted from person to person [1 – 2]. Annually, 100 million cases of dengue fever and half a million cases of DHF occur worldwide [27]. An infected female Aedes mosquito transmits the virus from person to person while feeding. Generally, the Aedes mosquito is usually most active in the early morning after daybreak, in the late afternoon before dark and anytime during the day when indoors or in shady areas [1 – 2]. The classical form of this infection resembles viral flu: fever, headache, chill and rash. Most of affected patients have a complete recovery without any complication [28 – 30]. Dengue fever is rarely fatal. However, there is a severe form of dengue infection called dengue hemorrhagic fever (DHF). In this case, several host immunological responses including immune complex formation, complement activation, increased histamine release and a massive release of many cytokines into the circulation, are the important factors in the course of disease [31]. Ninety percent of DHF subjects are children less than 15 years of age [27]. Also, DHF is an important cause of childhood death in many tropical countries [27].

Although dengue fever is found mostly in Asia, Africa and the Caribbean, in the recent year many American cases were confirmed to have contracted the disease [1 – 2]. At present, dengue is endemic in 112 countries in the world [27]. The important of traveling medicine is noted in this case. The lapse in mosquito eradication programs and the increase of unplanned urbanization, resulting in large populations living with inadequate systems of water and solid waste management, allowed the Aedes species to find excellent breeding places [1 – 2]. Guzman and Kouri recently said that the epidemiological situation in Latin America resembled that in Southeast Asia. They noted that during 2002, more than 30 Latin American countries reported over 1000000 dengue fever cases and DHF occurred in 20 countries with more than 17000 DHF cases, including 225 fatalities [32]. In addition, they reported that the co-circulation of multiple serotypes has been reported from many countries [32]. Conclusively, Guzman and Kouri mentioned that in the Americas, DHF was observed both in children and adults; secondary infection by a different dengue virus serotype had been confirmed as an important risk factor for this severe form of the disease, however, some new risk factors such as the interval of dengue virus infections and the ethnicity and underlying chronic conditions of the patient had also been identified [32]. They also concluded that the sequence of dengue virus infections and association with certain genotypes were further factors of importance [32].

Although infection with dengue stimulates immunologic response to a serotype, there is no cross-immunity conferred [33]. Hence, a person can potentially be infected with each serotype during his or her lifetime [33]. Castleberry and Mahon mentioned that because of the major impact on lives and local economies epidemics produce, rapid detection of dengue infection had become an important public health research issue [33]. They also noted that recently developed serological procedures to detect dengue infections had shown great potential for field use [33]. Dengue diagnosis was one of the topics discussed at the symposium 'The Global Threat of Dengue - Desperately Seeking Solutions' organized during the 10th International Congress of Infectious Diseases held in Singapore in 2002 [34]. Guzman and Kouri noted that IgM capture ELISA, virus isolation in mosquito cell lines and live mosquitoes, dengue specific monoclonal antibodies and PCR had all represented major advances in dengue diagnosis, however, an appropriate rapid, early and accessible diagnostic method useful both for epidemiological surveillance and clinical diagnosis was still needed [34]. Guzman and Kouri also said that laboratory infrastructure, technical expertise and research capacity must be improved in endemic countries in order to positively influence dengue surveillance, clinical case management and the development of new approaches to dengue control [34].Generally, dengue fever can be resolve without specific treatment. Some supportive treatment such as bed rest, fluids and fever medications are recommended [28 - 29]. Occasionally, as already mentioned, the disease can progress into DHF, a more serious illness with several abnormal bleeding presentations [35]. In the cases with DHF, dengue shock syndrome, a very low blood pressure, is a totally unwanted complication. The prevention of this disease is avoiding the mosquito bite. Until present, no vaccine is available for preventing this disease [27]. Malavige *et al* said that early recognition and prompt initiation of appropriate treatment were vital if disease related morbidity and mortality were to be limited [27].

D. Encephalitis Due t Mosquito-Borne Viral Infection

Viral encephalitis occurs in epidemic settings or is sporadic. Human infections by encephalitis viruses are usually asymptomatic or symptoms are not specific to these viruses. Encephalitis due to mosquito-borne viral infection is an important group of mosquito-borne diseases [36]. New encephalitis patterns reflect the roles that biologic reservoirs and vectors play in determining virus-human interactions [37]. Because these diseases are frequent in developing countries and tend to emerge or re-emerge in others, diagnostic tools must detect the broadest possible range of viruses with a high sensitivity and this is a key factor for surveillance, control of transmission and prevention through vaccination [36]. In addition, in countries with limited diagnostic infrastructures, low-cost and easy-to-use tests are required [36]. There are several mosquito-borne viral encephalitis. Some of those are presented as the followings:

West Nile Viral Encephalitis

West Nile (WN) virus is a mosquito-borne flavivirus and human, equine, and avian neuropathogen. Indeed, the West Nile virus is a form of encephalitis, a generic term for the inflammation of the brain caused by bacterial or viral infections [37]. It has been responsible for millions of human infections from the Western Mediterranean and Africa through the Middle East [37]. West Nile virus encephalitis has emerged in the Western hemisphere after apparent abrupt translocation of this mosquito-borne virus to a distant geographic region with immunologically naive avian and human hosts [37]. In 1996 the West Nile virus spread into Europe and in 1999 it was found in New York City [1 – 2]. Harrison noted that After the New York outbreak of West Nile Virus encephalitis in the summer of 1999, awareness that vulnerable children and adolescents might be at risk for this mosquito-borne viral infection intensified [38]. During 1999-2002, the virus extended its range throughout much of the eastern parts of the USA [39]. During 1999-2001, 142 cases of neuroinvasive WN viral disease of the central nervous system (including 18 fatalities), and seven cases of uncomplicated WN fever were reported in the USA [39].

One of the most common mosquitoes, the Culex species, is known to carry the West Nile virus [1 – 2]. Birds are the natural hosts for the West Nile virus, transmitting the disease to humans and other animals through the bites of infected mosquitoes [1 – 2]. Therefore, the Wile Nile encephalitis is also considered as an important zoonosis. Microbiologically, WN is an RNA virus and a member of the Flaviviridae family [40]. As previously mentioned, the main hosts are birds and the principle vectors are mosquitoes, usually of the genus Culex

[40]. Crook *et al* noted that while a few human cases have been identified in returning travelers, WN virus has not been reported in any animal or bird in the UK [40]. They noted that potential avian hosts and mosquito vectors of WN virus were present in the UK and birds migrated to the UK from areas of endemic WN virus activity [40]. They also noted that the population density of mosquitoes was relatively low and therefore the risk of WNV being transmitted in the UK was thought to be low [40].

Symptoms of the disease begin three to 12 days following a bite from an infected mosquito [39]. Most human WN viral infections are subclinical but clinical infections can range in severity from uncomplicated WN fever to fatal meningoencephalitis [39]. Although most infected people do not become symptomatic, severe diseases such as encephalitis and, less commonly, aseptic meningitis may occur, more frequently in the elderly [40]. Early symptoms include fever, headache, body aches, drowsiness, vomiting, a skin rash and swollen lymph glands [39 – 40]. More severe cases can cause high fever, focal paralysis, disorientation, coma, convulsions and death [39 – 40]. Young children, adults over the age of 50 and individuals with weak immune systems are more at risk for severe infections. Campbell *et al* concluded that the incidence of severe neuroinvasive disease and death increase with age [39]. Crook *et al* noted that clinicians were advised to consider WN virus as a differential diagnosis, especially in patients over 50 years old with a clinical picture of viral encephalitis or aseptic meningitis presenting in the summer months [40]. Concerning the diagnosis, serology remains the mainstay of laboratory diagnostic test [39 – 41]. Until present, no WN virus-specific treatment or vaccine is available [39 – 41]. Prevention depends on organised, sustained vector mosquito control, and public education [39 – 41]. Crook *et al* recently proposed that the public could be protected by giving advice on the avoidance of mosquito bites and by the implementation of ecological surveillance and measures to reduce the mosquito population [40].

Japanese Viral Encephalitis

Japanese encephalitis (JE) virus is a mosquito-borne flavivirus that can cause encephalitis and death in horses and humans [42 – 43]. It is an emerging disease of international concern because it has been spreading into previously nonendemic areas [42 – 43]. Ellis *et al* noted that major epidemics might occur where the virus moves into new areas, but many infections were subclinical [42 – 43]. Tiroumourougane *et al* noted that one of the leading causes of acute encephalopathy in children in the tropics was Japanese encephalitis [43]. This virus can be transmitted by the culex mosquito [42 – 43]. Pathophysiologically, this neurotropic virus predominately affects the thalamus, anterior horns of the spinal cord, cerebral cortex, and cerebellum [43]. Generally, it mainly affects children under 15 years and is mostly asymptomatic [42 – 43]. Clinically, the patient who either resides in an endemic region or who has been exposed to the viral vector, the mosquito, may have symptoms including high fever, headache, and impaired consciousness [44]. The occasional symptomatic child typically presents with a neurological syndrome characterised by altered sensorium, seizures, and features of intracranial hypertension [42- 43]. As already mentioned, the pathology of encephalitism involves many portions of the supratentorial and infratentorial compartments including the brain stem, hippocampus, thalamus, basal ganglia, and white matter [44].

Etiological diagnosis is based on virus isolation or demonstration of virus specific antigen or antibodies in the cerebrospinal fluid/blood [43]. Radiologically, MR imaging demonstrates the lesions of JE as hyperintense on T2-weighted images and hypointense on T1-weighted images [44]. Abe *et al* noted that Hemorrhagic transformations have also been described in JE lesions, with corresponding expected T1 and T2 changes [44]. Abe *et al* also noted that differential considerations based on the MRI appearance are somewhat broad, including but not limited to primary viral encephalitis, acute encephalopathy, limbic encephalitis, and acute disseminated encephalomyelitis [44]. The therapy for this viral encephalitis is primarily conservative and supportive since there is no specific treatment, and the disease has a high fatality rate [44]. The prognosis depends on the extent of involvement at primary presentation, and on the autoimmune mechanisms of this disease [44]. Though no antiviral drug is available against JE, effective supportive management can improve the outcome [43]. Control of JE involves efficient vector control and appropriate use of vaccines [43].

St. Louis Encephalitis

Arboviruses are important considerations in the differential diagnosis of encephalitis and other acute infections. Tsai noted that alterations in the environment and in human behaviors contributed to changing patterns of arboviral transmission and these trends, the periodic epidemic resurgence of arboviral diseases such as St. Louis encephalitis [45]. The St. Louis encephalitis virus is found throughout North, Central, and South America, and the Caribbean, but is a major public health problem in the United States [1 – 2]. Concerning the infection, the elderly and the young are most at risk and upto 30 percent of elderly patients infected with the virus will die [46].

One of the species of mosquitoes known to carry the St. Louis encephalitis virus is the Culex species [46]. Of interest, this infection cannot be transmitted from person-to-person or animal-to-person [46]. In 1980 Reeves wrote that epidemics of St. Louis encephalitis were preventable by means of surveillance and vector abatement [47]. Reeves described that 5 interactive factors (virus, vector, viremic host, human immunity, environmental temperature) are important for epidemic [47]. Monath and Tsai noted that although much progress has been achieved, many questions remain about St. Louis Encephalitis epidemiology and ecology [47].

Clinically, symptoms of the disease begin five to fifteen days after being bit but most individuals never show any outward symptoms [46]. Mild cases include flu-like symptoms, with fever, headaches and lethargy [46]. Similar to other viral encephalitis, severe cases of the virus can cause seizures, double vision, paralysis and death [46].

Rift Valley Fever

Rift Valley fever virus is an arthropod-borne Phlebovirus endemic in sub-Saharan Africa [48]. Outbreaks also have occurred in Egypt, Madagascar, and most recently in the Arabian peninsula [48]. Large epizootics occur at irregular intervals in seasons of above-average rainfall with persistent flooding and the appearance of large numbers of floodwater-breeding

Aedes mosquitoes [48]. The virus is transmitted transovarially and can remain dormant in mosquito eggs during dry interepizootic periods [48].

Rift Valley fever can affect both animals and humans. In animal, Rift Valley Fever is characterized by abortion in pregnant animals and a high mortality in newborn lambs, kids, and calves [48]. In humans, Rift Valley fever is a zoonosis, and human beings experience an influenza-like illness and, more rarely, complications such as encephalitis or retinitis [48 - 49]. Although Rift Valley fever presents as a flu-like disease but occasionally leads to high morbidity and mortality [48 – 49]. For humans, the disease is generally known in the African continent [49]. However, cases started to appear in Middle East including Saudi Arabia and Yemen [49]. Diagnosis is based on histopathology or the demonstration of viral antigen or antibody [48]. This new emerging disease should be concern from all physicians.

MAGNITUDE OF TROPICAL MOSQUITO-BORNE DISEASES

Mosquito-borne disease is considered to be a common public health problem worldwide. The tropical mosquito-borne diseases show similar high prevalence in each tropical region of the world, however, there might be difference in types of disorders. Here, the summary of reports concerning the magnitude and patterns of tropical mosquito-borne diseases in many tropical regions is presented.

- South Asia

Mosquito-borne diseases are important public health problem to many countries in South Asia. In 2003, Snehalatha *et al* studied the mosquito problem in South India. In that study, the severity of mosquito nuisance and the type and costs of personal protection measures in the Pondicherry region had been investigated, using a structured questionnaire [50]. According to this study, 87 and 63% of the urban and rural respondents, respectively, felt that mosquito nuisance was severe in their locality [50]. In addition, 83% of the urban and 27% of the rural respondents were aware that mosquitoes transmit diseases and were able to name at least one mosquito-borne disease [50].

In Pakistan, Mosquito breeding within the wastewater irrigation system around the town of Haroonabad in the southern Punjab, Pakistan, was recently studied by Mukhtar *et al* [51]. According to this study, wastewater disposal and irrigation systems provided a perennial source of water for vector mosquitos in semi-arid countries like Pakistan [51]. Overall, 17.3% of the samples were positive for Anopheles, 12.0% for Culex and 15.0% for Aedes [51]. Mukhtar *et al* concluded that vector mosquitos exploited these sites if alternative breeding sites with better biological, physical, and chemical conditions were not abundant [51].

There was also another interesting report from Bangladesh [52]. Birley reviewed the evidence of a link between flood control and vector-borne disease in Bengal/Bangladesh [68]. Birley found that malaria was historically associated with reduced flooding and embankment construction in the flood plains of Bengal [52].

Birley also noted that Bancroftian filariasis had a widespread but usually low prevalence in Bangladesh, with both rural and urban foci and increasing organic pollution and drainage obstruction are expected to favour the vector and increase transmission [52].

- West Asia

Indeed, some non-mosquito arthropod-borne diseases such as leishmaniasis and trypanosomiasis are common in the Middle East. The explanation might be related to the dry weather, which is not proper for breeding of mosquitoes. However, malaria still exists in this area. There are some interesting reports concerning the prevalence of mosquito-borne diseases in West Asia. An entomological surveillance was conducted in Asir, Jizan, and Makkah regions, Kingdom of Saudi Arabia in response to a recent outbreak of Rift Valley fever [53]. According to this study, the first record of *Aedes unilineatus* in Arabian Peninsula was reported [53].

- Southeast Asia

In Southeast Asia, the mosquitoes are common in both rural and urban areas [54]. Therefore, the mosquito-borne diseases are also common. The two common mosquito-borne diseases in this area are malaria and dengue fever. It is proposed that all human malarial parasites originated from zoonotic simian plasmodiids in tropical forests of southeastern Asia, during the terminal Pleistocene or early Holocene [55]. The modes of malarial transmission among prehistoric natives of that geographic area are reconstructed, based primarily on ecological, archeological and ethnographic evidence [55]. Poolsuwan noted that with the abundance and interactive roles in transmitting human malaria of the *Anopheles dirus* and *Anopheles minimus* mosquitos in forest fringe areas, the middle Holocene settled farmers occupying such habitats would have been subject all year round to highly endemic malaria [55]. Poolsuwan also mentioned that much lower and less uniform transmission of the disease could have been found among early coastal occupants, in the presence of the less efficient *Anopheles sundaicus* vector [55]. Kondrashin and Rooney said that varying host-parasite-vector interrelationships are shown to be influenced significantly by prevailing environmental conditions as well as behavioral and socio-economic determinants [56]. Kondrashin and Rooney also mentioned that drug-resistant falciparum malaria and vector resistance to insecticides were the main biological deterrents to the success of control programs, therefore, the potential for malaria transmission remained high in many places [56]. They suggested that malaria control strategy should include Primary Health Care and integration with basic health services [56].

Dengue Fever and DHF have been the most common urban diseases in Southeast Asia since the 1950s [57]. Both Aedes aegypti and Aedes albopictus are involved in the transmission of dengue fever /DHF in Southeast Asian region [57]. Recently Yap *et al* mentioned for the vector control approaches which include source reduction and environmental management, larviciding with the use of chemicals (synthetic insecticides and insect growth regulators and microbial insecticide), and adulticiding which include personal protection measures (household insecticide products and repellents) for long-term control and space spray (both thermal fogging and ultra low volume sprays) as short-term epidemic measures [57]. In this article, the advantages of using water-based spray over the oil-based spray and the use of spray formulation which provide both larvicidal and adulticidal effects that would consequently have greater impact on the overall vector and disease control in dengue fever/DHF are highlighted [57].

Filariasis is a less common mosquito-borne disease in the Southeast Asia. Mak noted that the distribution and transmission of the disease were closely associated with socioeconomic and behavioural factors in endemic populations [58]. Mak said that Urban *Wuchereria bancrofti* infection, as seen in South-East Asia, was related to poor urban sanitation, which led to intense breeding of *Culex quiquefasciatus*, the principal vector [58].

- Latin America

The mosquito-borne diseases are common in the Latin America. Dengue infection constitutes one of the most rapidly expanding and re-emerging infectious disease problems in Latin America [59]. In less than 20 years, the region has transformed itself from hypoendemic to hyperendemic, while serotype circulation in most countries has gone from none or single to multiple [59]. Isturiz *et al* said that Health care providers who see patients in or returning from areas of Latin America, the Caribbean, and other tropical areas must consider dengue in the differential diagnosis of patients presenting with compatible symptoms, and must be knowledgeable in the current management of this important disease [59].

Concerning malaria, Singer and de Castro said that land use patterns, linked to social organization of the community and the structure of the physical environment, played a key role in promoting malaria transmission on the Amazon frontier [76]. In addition, the location of each occupied area was itself an important determinant of the pattern of malaria risk [60].

Yellow fever is still present at Latin America. Outbreaks of yellow fever in recent years in the South America have prompted concern about the possible urbanization of jungle fever [61]. Recently said that yellow fever endemicity was stabilized in South America: an average of 115 cases has officially been notified each year since 25 years [62]. They said that yellow fever definitely remains a topical disease, which required a constant surveillance [62]. Monath noted that since residents of the densely populated cities and much visited areas in coastal South America had never been vaccinated, an outbreak there would facilitate widespread dissemination of the disease, even to other continents [63]. Isturiz *et al* concluded that malaria, cholera, typhoid fever, yellow fever are the important problem for the travelers visiting Latin America [64].

- Africa

Africa can been mentioned as the area with the highest poverty in the world. Several tropical diseases are endemic in Africa. In 1995, Guyatt and Snow performed a meatanalysis for eighteen studies from areas with stable malaria transmission in sub-Saharan Africa and found that the median prevalence of severe anemia in all-parity pregnant women was approximately 8.2% [65]. They proposed that if assumed that 26% of these cases were due to malaria, it had been suggested that as many as 400,000 pregnant women might have developed severe anemia as a result of infection with malaria in sub-Saharan Africa [65].

Concerning dengue infection, *Aedes aegypti* is believed to be originated from Africa and expanded around the tropical world [66]. However, the dengue infection in less common than Southeast Asia, the original of denuge [67 - 68]. Yellow fever, present in Africa mostly in restricted areas [67]. In the last 25 years of the 20th century, however, there was a resurgence of yellow fever in Africa, and of dengue worldwide [67]. The other viral mosquito-borne diseases are also detected in Africa. Of several viral diseases, West Nile virus infection is the well known viral mosquito-borne disease with the long history from Africa [37].

Some present concerns on Tropical Mosquito-Borne Diseases

1. Mosquito-Borne Disease in Non-Tropical Countries

The existence of mosquito-borne diseases in many non-tropical countries is considered an important public heath problem at present. These diseases are considered as an important emerging infectious problem in the Western hemisphere. Lundstrom said that several mosquito-borne arboviruses belonging to the genera Alphavirus, Flavivirus, and Bunyavirus have been reported to occur in mosquitoes and to infect humans and other vertebrates in Western Europe [69]. Lundstrom proposed that specific sampling of potential vectors for virus isolation, detailed characterization of virus strains, and the use of fully characterized strains for serological diagnosis would help to elucidate the present and future potential of mosquito-borne viruses as human pathogens in Europe [69].

Concerning flaviviruses –related mosquito-borne disease, Mackenzie *et al* recently described three of them: the resurgence of dengue in tropical and subtropical areas of the world, and the spread and establishment of Japanese encephalitis and West Nile viruses in new habitats and environments [70]. They said that these three examples also illustrate the complexity of the various factors that contributed to their emergence, resurgence and spread [70]. They noted that whereas some of these factors are natural, such as bird migration, most are due to human activities, such as changes in land use, water impoundments and transportation, which resulted in changed epidemiological patterns [70]. Finally Mackenzie *et al* concluded that the three examples also show the ease with which mosquito-borne viruses could spread to and colonize new areas, and the need for continued international surveillance and improved public health infrastructure to meet future emerging disease threats [70].

The possible factors contributing to the changing in the epidemiology of tropical mosquito-borne diseases from tropical to non tropical zone include the good transportation system, travelling and tourism, urbanization, mutation of the pathogens and the changing of environmental temperature as mentioned as the "Global Warming").

2. Uncommon Modes of Transmission of Tropical Mosquito-Borne Diseases

Some tropical mosquito-borne diseases have addition modes of transmission to vector transmission. Malaria is a good example. This infection can be transmitted via blood and placental transfusion. Concerning the West Nile virus infection, it is also considered as a zoonosis. To control of these diseases, the public health care worker must concern these uncommon modes of transmissions as well.

3. Co-Occurrence of Tropical Mosquito-Borne Diseases

The co-occurrence of tropical mosquito-borne diseases can be seen and is usually a difficult – to - treat condition in medicine. A good example is a cooccurrence between falciparum and vivax malaria [71 - 72]. Recently Mason andMcKenzie performed a mathematical model study and suggested several phenomena that might merit clinical attention, including the potential recrudescence of a long-standing, low-level *Plasmodium falciparum* infection following a *Plasmodium vivax* infection or relapse and the capacity of an existing *Plasmodium vivax* infection to reduce the peak parasitemia of a *Plasmodium falciparum* superinfection [73]. They also simulated the administration of antimalarial drugs, and illustrate some potential complications in treating mixed-species malaria infections and they found that when a mixed-species infection is misdiagnosed as a single-species *Plasmodium vivax* infection, treatment for *Plasmodium vivax* can lead to a surge in *Plasmodium falciparum* parasitemia [73].

REFERENCES

[1] Vector borne diseases. Available at http://www.fpnotebook.com/ID211.htm
[2] Changes in the Incidence of Vector-Borne Diseases Attributable to Climate Change. Available at http://www.ciesin.org/TG/HH/veclev2.html
[3] Schlagenhauf P. Malaria: from prehistory to present. *Infect Dis Clin North Am*. 2004; 18: 189-205.
[4] Green AD, Roberts KI. Recent trends in infectious diseases for travellers. *Occup Med (Lond)*. 2000; 50: 560-5.
[5] Suyaphun A, Wiwanitkit V, Suwansaksri J, Nithiuthai S, Sritar S, Suksirisampant W, Fongsungnern A. Malaria among hilltribe communities in northern Thailand: a review of clinical manifestations. *Southeast Asian J Trop Med PublicHealth*. 2002; 33 Suppl 3: 14-5.
[6] Mazzarello P, Calligaro AL. Golgi's documents about the history of malaria. *Med Secoli*. 1998; 10: 495-510.
[7] Reiter P. From Shakespeare to Defoe: malaria in England in the Little Ice Age. *Emerg Infect Dis*. 2000; 6: 1-11.
[8] Dobson MJ. History of malaria in England. *J R Soc Med*. 1989; 82 Suppl 17: 3-7.
[9] Carcaterra P. Rome and malaria. *Med Secoli*. 1998; 10: 557-77.
[10] Bruce-Chwatt LJ. The social history of malaria in Europe. *Soc Hist Med Bull*. (Lond). 1978; (1):17-18.
[11] Wiwanitkit V. Amazing Thailand Year 1998-1999 Tourist's health concepts. *Chula Med J*. 1998; 43: 975-984.
[12] Julvez J. History of insular malaria in the southwestern Indian Ocean: an eco-epidemiologic approach. *Sante*. 1995; 5: 353-8.
[13] Najera JA. Malaria control: achievements, problems and strategies. *Parassitologia*. 2001; 43: 1-89.
[14] Lawrence RA. Lymphatic filariasis: What mice can tell us. *Parasitol Today*. 1996; 12: 267-71.
[15] Kimmig P, Hassler D. Filaria of the lymphatic system: Wuchereria, Brugia. *Dtsch Med Wochenschr*. 2004; 129: 1493-4.
[16] Ottesen EA, Ramachandran CP. Lymphatic filariasis infection and disease: control strategies. *Parasitology Today*. 1995; 11: 129 –31.
[17] Hoerauf A. Control of filarial infections: not the beginning of the end, but more research is needed. *Curr Opin Infect Dis*. 2003; 16: 403-10.

[18] Dreyer G, Noroes J, Figueredo-Silva J, Piessens WF. Pathogenesis of lymphatic disease in bancroftian filariasis: a clinical perspective. *Parasitol Today*. 2000; 16: 544-8.
[19] Walther M, Muller R. Diagnosis of human filariases (except onchocerciasis). *Adv Parasitol.* 2003; 53:149-93.
[20] Wiwanitkit V. Prevaelnce of filariasis in Myanmar migrant workers in Bangsaparn district, Prachuab Kiri Khan province Thailand. Presented at the Joint international Tropical Medicine Meeting 2001. Bangkok: Thailand, 2001
[21] Triteeraprapab S. Update in lymphatic filariasis: A re-emerging disease of Thailand. *Chula Med J.* 1996; 41: 611 – 22.
[22] Triteeraprapab S, Songtrus J. High prevalence of Bancroftian filariasis in Myanamar-migrant workers: a study in Mae Sot District, Tak Province, Thailand. *J Med Assoc Thai.* 1999; 82: 734 – 9.
[23] Chaipet S. Lymphatic filariasis. *Thai. Malaria. J.* 1982; 27: 61 – 71.
[24] Richard-Lenoble D, Chandenier J, Gaxotte P. Ivermectin and filariasis. *Fundam Clin Pharmacol.* 2003; 17: 199-203.
[25] Wiwanitkit V. Wolbachia infection in filarial nematodes, new trend in the study on macrofilaricides. *Songklanagarind Med J.* 2001; 19: 235 – 9.
[26] Thisyakorn U, Thisyakorn C. Diseases caused by arboviruses-dengue hemorrhagic fever and Japanese B encephalitits. *Med J Aus*. 1994; 160: 22 – 26.
[27] Malavige GN, Fernando S, Fernando DJ, Seneviratne SL. Dengue viral infections. *Postgrad Med J.* 2004; 80: 588-601.
[28] Guzman MG, Kouri G. Dengue: an update. *Lancet Infect Dis*. 2002; 2: 33-42.
[29] da Fonseca BA, Fonseca SN. Dengue virus infections. *Curr Opin Pediatr*. 2002; 14: 67-711.
[30] Solomon T, Mallewa M. Dengue and other emerging flaviviruses. *J Infect*. 2001; 42:104-15.
[31] Mitrakul C. Bleeding problem in dengue haemorrhagic fever: platelets and coagulation changes. *Southeast Asian J Trop Med Public Health*. 1987; 18: 407-412.
[32] Guzman MG, Kouri G. Dengue and dengue hemorrhagic fever in the Americas: lessons and challenges. *J Clin Virol*. 2003; 27:1-13.
[33] Castleberry JS, Mahon CR. Dengue fever in the Western Hemisphere. *Clin Lab Sci.* 2003; 16: 34-8.
[34] Guzman MG, Kouri G. Dengue diagnosis, advances and challenges. *Int J Infect Dis*. 2004; 8: 69-80.
[35] Wiwanitkit V. Bleeding and other presentations in Thai patients with dengue infection. *Clin Appl Thromb Hemost.* 2004; 10: 397-8.
[36] Vernet G. Diagnosis of zoonotic viral encephalitis. *Arch Virol Suppl*. 20004; (18): 231-44.
[37] McCarthy M. Newer viral encephalitides. *Neurologist*. 2003; 9: 189-99.
[38] Harrison TW. West Nile encephalitis. *J Pediatr Health Care.* 2002; 16: 278-81.
[39] Campbell GL, Marfin AA, Lanciotti RS, Gubler DJ. West Nile virus. *Lancet Infect Dis*. 2002; 2: 519-29.
[40] Crook PD, Crowcroft NS, Brown DW. West Nile virus and the threat to the UK. Commun *Dis Public Health*. 2002; 5: 138-43.

[41] Katz LH, Brenner B, Robenshtok E, Ankol OH, Green MS, Hourvitz A, Weinberger M. West Nile fever: the virus, the mosquito, the disease and our coping. *Harefuah*. 2002; 141: 532-7.
[42] Ellis PM, Daniels PW, Banks DJ. Japanese encephalitis. *Vet Clin North Am Equine Pract.* 2002; 16: 565-78.
[43] Tiroumourougane SV, Raghava P, Srinivasan S. Japanese viral encephalitis. *Postgrad Med J.* 2002; 78: 205-15.
[44] Abe T, Kojima K, Shoji H, Tanaka N, Fujimoto K, Uchida M, Nishimura H, Hayabuchi N, Norbash AM. Japanese encephalitis. *J Magn Reson Imaging*. 1998; 8: 755-61.
[45] Tsai TF. Arboviral infections in the United States. *Infect Dis Clin North Am*. 1991; 5: 73-102.
[46] Ruby JP. St. Louis encephalitis. *Epidemiol Rev*. 1979; 1: 55-73.
[47] Monath TP, Tsai TF. St. Louis encephalitis: lessons from the last decade. *Am J Trop Med Hyg*. 1987; 37(3 Suppl): 40S-59S.
[48] Gerdes GH. Rift valley fever. *Vet Clin North Am Food Anim Pract*. 2002; 18: 549-55.
[49] Shawky S. Rift valley fever. *Saudi Med J.* 2000; 21: 1109-15.
[50] Snehalatha KS, Ramaiah KD, Vijay Kumar KN, Das PK. The mosquito problem and type and costs of personal protection measures used in rural and urban communities in Pondicherry region, South India. *Acta Trop*. 2003; 88: 3-9.
[51] Mukhtar M, Herrel N, Amerasinghe FP, Ensink J, van der Hoek W, Konradsen F. Role of wastewater irrigation in mosquito breeding in south Punjab, Pakistan. *Southeast Asian J Trop Med Public Health*. 2003; 34: 72-80.
[52] Birley MH. An historical review of malaria, kala-azar and filariasis in Bangladesh in relation to the Flood Action Plan. *Ann Trop Med Parasitol*. 1993; 87: 319-34.
[53] Godsey MS Jr, Abdoon AM, Savage HM, Al-Sharani AM, Al-Mazrou Y, Al-Jeffri MH, Al-Sughair S, Al-Safi S, Ksiazek TG, Miller BR. First record of Aedes (Stegomyia) unilineatus in the Kingdom of Saudi Arabia. *J Am Mosq Control Assoc*. 2003; 19: 84-6.
[54] Bang YH, Shah NK. Human ecology related to urban mosquito-borne diseases in countries of South East Asia region. *J Commun Dis*. 1988; 20: 1-17.
[55] Poolsuwan S. Malaria in prehistoric southeastern Asia. *Southeast Asian J Trop Med Public Health.* 1995; 26: 3-22.
[56] Kondrashin AV, Rooney W. Overview: epidemiology of malaria and its control in countries of the WHO South-East Asia region. *Southeast Asian J Trop Med Public Health*. 1992; 23 Suppl 4:13-22.
[57] Yap HH, Chong NL, Foo AE, Lee CY. Dengue vector control: present status and future prospects. *Gaoxiong Yi Xue Ke Xue Za Zhi*. 1987; 10 Suppl: S102-8.
[58] Mak JW. Epidemiology of lymphatic filariasis. *Ciba Found Symp*. 1987; 127: 5-14.
[59] Isturiz RE, Gubler DJ, Brea del Castillo J. Dengue and dengue hemorrhagic fever in Latin America and the Caribbean. *Infect Dis Clin North Am*. 2000; 14: 121-40.
[60] Singer BH, de Castro MC. Agricultural colonization and malaria on the Amazon frontier. *Ann NY Acad Sci*. 2001; 954: 184-222.
[61] Yellow fever vaccination in the Americas. *Bull Pan Am Health Organ*. 1984; 18: 188-92.
[62] Chippaux A, Deubel V, Moreau JP, Reynes JM. Current situation of yellow fever in Latin America. *Bull Soc Pathol Exot*. 1993; 86(5 Pt 2),460-4.
[63] Monath TP. Facing up to re-emergence of urban yellow fever. *Lancet*. 1999; 353: 1541.

[64] Isturiz RE, Stamboulian D, Lepetic A, Mondolfi A. Health advice for travelers to Latin America. *Infect Dis Clin North Am*. 1994; 8: 155-81.

[65] Guyatt HL, Snow RW. The epidemiology and burden of Plasmodium falciparum-related anemia among pregnant women in sub-Saharan Africa. *Am J Trop Med Hyg*. 2001;64(1-2 Suppl):36-44.

[66] Rodhain F. Ecology of Aedes aegypti in Africa and Asia. *Bull Soc Pathol Exot*. 1996; 89: 103-6.

[67] Gubler DJ. The changing epidemiology of yellow fever and dengue, 1900 to 2003: full circle? *Comp. Immunol Microbiol Infect Dis*. 2004; 27: 319-30.

[68] Zeller HG. Dengue, arbovirus and migrations in the Indian Ocean. *Bull Soc Pathol Exot*. 1998; 91: 56-60.

[69] Lundstrom JO. Mosquito-borne viruses in western Europe: a review. *J Vector Ecol*. 1999; 24:1-39.

[70] Mackenzie JS, Gubler DJ, Petersen LR. Emerging flaviviruses: the spread and resurgence of Japanese encephalitis, West Nile and dengue viruses. *Nat Med*. 2004; 10(12 Suppl): S98-S109.

[71] Snounou G, White NJ. The co-existence of Plasmodium: sidelights from falciparum and vivax malaria in Thailand. *Trends Parasitol*. 20, 333-9 (2004)

[72] Mayxay M, Pukrittayakamee S, Newton PN, White NJ. Mixed-species malaria infections in humans. *Trends Parasitol*. 2004; 20: 233-40.

[73] Mason DP, McKenzie FE. Blood-stage dynamics and clinical implications of mixed Plasmodium vivax-Plasmodium falciparum infections. *Am J Trop Med Hyg*. 1999; 61: 367-74.

Chapter 2

MALARIA IN GOLDEN TRIANGLE

ABSTRACT

Golden Triangle is a famous area of Southeast Asia. It is a triangle between Thailand, Myanmar and Laos. In this area, there are numerous hilltribers. Also, it is considered as an area with high public health and social problems. In this article, the situation and items relating to malaria in golden triangle will be discussed.

INTRODUCTION TO GOLDEN TRIANGLE

Golden Triangle is a famous area of Southeast Asia. It is a triangle between Thailand, Myanmar and Laos. In this area, there are numerous hilltribers. Also, it is considered as an area with high public health and social problems. It is the area with the highest problem of opium production. Heroin epidemics developed in most SA countries in the 1960s and early 1970s and remained a significant problem [1] Luckily, opium production has been illegal in Thailand since 1959 due to a highly successful crop substitution program undertaken by the Royal Projects Foundation established by His Majesty King Bhumipol, opium production has largely been eliminated in Thailand. However, across the border in Burma, the Shan United Army, which is fighting the central Burmese government for an independent Shan state, has been accused of funding its war through the sale of opium and heroin. Opiates, mainly opium and heroin, are the drugs of choice except in Thailand, where opiate abuse declined, but amphetamine is the main drug of abuse due to its low cost and availability [2]. Intravenous injection (IV) of drugs appeared after the heroin epidemic and currently prevails in countries with a significant opiate abuse problem. This problem can also lead to several consequence including AIDS and blood borne infectious diseases. According to the anthropologist opinion, the role of the drug abuse control team is to provide analyses of how development projects alter the social make-up of their target communities and contribute to ways in which substance use/abuse is understood, practiced and controlled or reconfigured [3]. Harm reduction can and should include pre-emptive concern with factors that promote damaging drug use in the first place and furthermore, that these factors are at times the products of the distinct drug reduction strategies themselves [3].

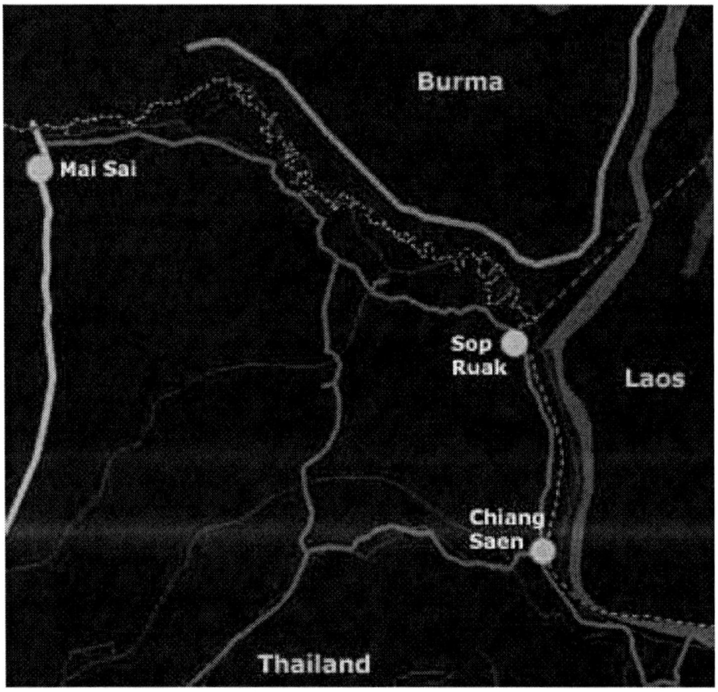

Figure 1. The area namely Sop Ruak, the heart of the Golden Triangle.

The Golden Triangle is a mountainous region, mostly covered by forest and inhabited by a tribal population estimated at 300,000 to 500,000 persons who live in some 3,000 villages [4 - 5]. The people, who are seminomadic move about with their personal property and weapons, without any form of control [4]. Many hilltribers in the distance areas have been cultivating the opium poppy since the beginning of the century and this single crop provides all that is needed for the livelihood of the families [4]. In additional to the problem of illegal drug, the Golden Triangle also poses several other public health problems. Many infectious diseases are still uncontrolled in the remote communities. Malaria is also highly prevalent here [4 – 6].

In this article, the situation and items relating to malaria in golden triangle will be discussed.

Important Problems of Malaria in the Golden Triangle

A. Malaria and Narcotic Drugs

Of interest, the problem of malaria and illegal opium coexist in the Golden Triangle. Malaria and opium control should be done on the parallel way [7]. Malaria surveillance is recommended for the increasing addict population in the cities of Southeast Asia [8]. The clustering of malaria infections among narcotic injectors who have not been in malarious areas indicates that the malaria is transmitted by the common use of needles and syringes [8 - 10]. Most of the cases are the patients with narcotic related malaria in the Western literature, who have occasionally abused heroin intravenously, shared injection equipment with an addict who had previously contracted malaria in Southeast Asia and who had failed to complete an adequate course of treatment [8 - 11]. The infection can be either vivax or falciparum malaria Cerebral malaria in an addict may be misdiagnosed as drug intoxication [8 - 14].

There are also some interesting features on the effect of narcotic on the pathophysiology of malaria. Singh reported that morphine exerted a dose-dependent, biphasic effect on the course of *Plasmodium berghei* infection in mice, apparently by modulating the macrophage-mediated protective mechanisms [15]. It was also reported that chloroquine could induce a severe generalized pruritus, in predisposed Black African patients, during treatment of malaria fever, and also in some Caucasian patients treated for rheumatological diseases [16]. Indeed, micro-opiate receptors/and or endogenous opioids may contribute to chloroquine itching in malaria fever, in humans, in accord with animal experimental findings [16]. In a rat model, opioidergic mechanisms can be confirmed [17]. It also strongly suggests that the chloroquine-induced body-scratching behavior in the rat may be a useful experimental model for chloroquine-induced pruritus in humans [17]. Ajayi proposed that malaria parasite density in blood was a strong determinant of itching severity in patients predisposed to chloroquine-induced pruritus [16].

B. Malaria and Hilltribers

Hilltribe is the main group of local population in the Golden Triangle [18]. These people are considered as an underprivileged group. There are six main ethnic groups among the hill tribe population: Karen, Hmong, Lahu, Akha, Yao, and H'tin [19]. Socioeconomic development in the villages is poor. The tribers think that evil spirits cause illness and do not seek care from a Western medical practitioner [20]. If they believe the illness was caused by natural causes, however, they do go to a medical practitioner [20]. Further, they believe vampires exist where many people are ill or dying and that the vampires will bite, so they are fearful of going to a hospital [20]. Tribal community is endemic for malaria. The risk factors included living or working in the forest, accompanying their family during movement through the forest, age < or =14 years, poor knowledge of how to protect against malaria, and unavailability of protection against malaria via long sleeved clothes, topical repellents, and insecticide treated nets (use and carry), which resulted in an increased exposure to malaria and risk for malaria infection [21]. Recently, Suyaphan et al reviewed the clinical manifestations presented by patients with malaria from the database of Mae Chaem Hospital, Chiang Mai Province. Mae Chaem district is hilly and rural. More than 80% of the district's population are members of hilltribes. The database showed that between July 2000 and April 2001, a final diagnosis of malaria was made in 94 cases. The commonest clinical manifestation was fever (96.8%), followed by chills (60.6%). Interestingly, some unusual presentations such as petechiae, abnormal menstruation, and jaundice were also found [22]. Hu et al performed another interesting study to evaluate the prevailing practice of presumptively diagnosing malaria in all cases of febrile illness in a clinic serving a refugee population on the Thai-Myanmar border and found that all cases offever should continue to be treated presumptively as malaria until laboratory facilities are made available [23].

EPIDEMIOLOGY OF MALARIA IN THE GOLDEN TRIANGLE AREA

Northern Thailand

The provinces with in the area of the Golden Triangle area of Thailand are the provinces in the North. Chiangmai and Chiangrai are the two mostfamous provinces. Locally, the malaria within the local people in this area can be successfully controlled. However, there are still the new cases from the migrant hill tribers from the nearby countries [24 – 25]. An interesting cross-sectional study was conducted from January, 2001 to June, 2002 among some migrant populations, living in malaria endemic areas along the Thai-Myanmar border, in the Mae Fah Luang and Mae Sai districts,Chiang Rai Province, Northern Thailand using blood exams and face-to-face interviews as the research methods [24]. According to this report, a poor knowledge of primary malaria prevention, the presence of international migration, poverty, lack of malaria prevention resources, namely bednets (not using or taking them) and not using a smoky fire were factors which led to failure in primary prevention and control of malaria infections [24].

Northwestern Laos

There are still limited numbers of researches on the malaria from the northern Laos. Local work is unavailable. However, there are some reports from the external researchers on the situation of malaria in this area. Dittrich et al studied the falciparum malaria in the north of Laos and found that the South American/PNG -haplotype (SVMNT) of Pfcrt-gene encodes a transmembrane protein located in the *P. falciparum* digestive vacuole could be detected [26]. Dittrich et al also proposed that distribution of the alleles showed significant differences between the north and the south province. Reasons for this include possible importation of different parasite strains from neighbouring countries [27].

Northeastern Myanmar

The area called Shan State in the northeastern Myanmar is still the area with a great difficulty to visit. The high prevalence of malaria in this area is expected, however, there is no exact data. Than et al reported that race was the dominant factor affecting the frequencies of red cell genetic disorders in malaria-endemic areas of Myanmar [28]. They demonstrated that abnormal hemoglobin variants and glucose-6-phosphate dehydrogenase (G6PD) deficiency were very high prevalent in this area [28]. Indeed, both malaria and hemoglobin E are endemic in this area of Myanmar indicating the important of natural selection process of malaria [29].

Southern China

Yunnan is the Southern-most area of China. There are also many hilltribers in Yunnan. An incidence of more than 10/10,000 distributing in Yunnan was reported according to the China database [30]. Yunnan still face a critical situation of malaria endemics with the spread of *P. falciparum*, especially in the border counties in Yunnan [30 - 31]. Of interest, the fifth species of human malaria, *P. knowlesi* infection, is firstly reported from malaria [32]. Concerning this type of malaria, ring forms had multinuclei, and the late trophozoites trended to form band [32]. The schizonts and gametocytes were somewhat alike to *P. vivax* [32].

Eastern India

Eastern India is the area next to the Golden Triangle. There are also many hilltribers in this area, especially in the state called Manipur. Singh et al reported that shows that knowledge regarding transmission of malaria, self protection and treatment seeking behavior is still poor among the tribal communities of Manipur [33]. However the urban tribals had better knowledge regarding diagnosis of malaria and prevention of mosquito breeding than their rural counterparts [33].

REFERENCES

[1] Poshyachinda V. Drugs and AIDS in Southeast-Asia. *Forensic Sci Int.* 1993;62:15-28.

[2] Kulsudjarit K. Drug problem in southeast and southwest Asia. *Ann N Y Acad Sci.* 2004 Oct;1025:446-57.

[3] Lyttleton C, Cohen PT. Harm reduction and alternative development in the Golden Triangle. *Drug Alcohol Rev.* 2003;22:83-91.

[4] Nepote J. In the golden triangle with a handful of dollars. *Bull Narc.* 1976;28:1-8.

[5] Kondrashin AV. Malaria in Southeast Asia. *Southeast Asian J Trop Med Public Health.* 1986;17:642-55.

[6] World malaria situation in 1990. *Bull World Health Organ.* 1992;70:801-4, 809-13.

[7] Rosa FW. Malaria and opium control in Iran. *Public Health Rep.* 1960;75:352-4.

[8] Brown JD, Khoa NQ. Fatal falciparum malaria among narcotic injectors. *Am J Trop Med Hyg.* 1975;24:729-33.

[9] Rosenblatt JE, Marsh VH. Induced malaria in narcotic addicts. *Lancet.* 1971;2:189-90.

[10] Colombo E, Gambelli F, Marchetti L, Sciariada L, Velati C, Mari E. Plasmodium falciparum malaria transmitted through human contact in a group of drug addicts. *Minerva Med.* 1982;73:3445-8.

[11] Baker JE, Crawford GP. Malaria: a new facet of heroin addiction in Australia. *Med J Aust.* 1978;2:427-8.

[12] Friedmann CT, Dover AS, Roberto RR, Kearns OA. A malaria epidemic among heroin users. *Am J Trop Med Hyg.* 1973;22:302-7.

[13] Lyman DO, Boese RJ, Shearer LA. Malaria among heroin users. *Health Serv Rep.* 1972;87:545-9.

[14] Louria DB. Infectious complications of nonalcoholic drug abuse. *Annu Rev Med.* 1974;25:219-31.
[15] Singh PP, Singh S, Dutta GP, Srimal RC. Immunomodulation by morphine in Plasmodium berghei-infected mice. *Life Sci.* 1994;54:331-9.
[16] Ajayi AA, Kolawole BA, Udoh SJ. Endogenous opioids, mu-opiate receptors and chloroquine-induced pruritus: a double-blind comparison of naltrexone and promethazine in patients with malaria fever who have an established history of generalized chloroquine-induced itching. *Int J Dermatol.* 2004;43:972-7.
[17] Onigbogi O, Ajayi AA, Ukponmwan OE. Mechanisms of chloroquine-induced body-scratching behavior in rats: evidence of involvement of endogenous opioid peptides. *Pharmacol Biochem Behav.* 2000;65:333-7.
[18] Vichitbandha P, Parnsingha T, Podhipleux P, Yongchaiyud S, Suchatanondh M, Vichitbandha C, Viseskul D, Jaroonvesama N, Hinjiranan S, Pemayon B, Kompayak C, Vajanaprichasiri P, Suksthit S, Bankeang C, Yongchiyud P, Petchareon S, Udomratana L, Na-ranong S, Lekumphon T. Problems of hilltribe people and integrated development. *J Med Assoc Thai.* 1981;64:159-73.
[19] Aguettant JL. Impact of population registration on hilltribe development in Thailand. *Asia Pac Popul J.* 1996;11:47-72.
[20] Taking education to the hills. *JOICFP News.* 1991;(208):7.
[21] Pichainarong N, Chaveepojnkamjorn W. Malaria infection and life-style factors among hilltribes along the Thai-Myanmar border area, northern Thailand. *Southeast Asian J Trop Med Public Health.* 2004;35:834-9.
[22] Suyaphun A, Wiwanitkit V, Suwansaksri J, Nithiuthai S, Sritar S, Suksirisampant W, Fongsungnern A. Malaria among hilltribe communities in northern Thailand: a review of clinical manifestations. *Southeast Asian J Trop Med Public Health.* 2002;33 Suppl 3:14-5.
[23] Hu KK, Maung C, Katz DL. Clinical diagnosis of malaria on the Thai-Myanmar border. *Yale J Biol Med.* 2001;74:303-8.
[24] Chaveepojnkamjorn W, Pichainarong N. Behavioral factors and malaria infection among the migrant population, Chiang Rai province. *J Med Assoc Thai.* 2005;88:1293-301.
[25] Chaveepojnkamjorn W, Pichainarong N. Malaria infection among the migrant population along the Thai-Myanmar border area. *Southeast Asian J Trop Med Public Health.* 2004;35:48-52.
[26] Dittrich S, Alifrangis M, Stohrer JM, Thongpaseuth V, Vanisaveth V, Phetsouvanh R, Phompida S, Khalil IF, Jelinek T. Falciparum malaria in the north of Laos: the occurrence and implications of the Plasmodium falciparum chloroquine resistance transporter (pfcrt) gene haplotype SVMNT. *Trop Med Int Health.* 2005;10:1267-70.
[27] Dittrich S, Schwobel B, Jordan S, Vanisaveth V, Rattanaxay P, Christophel EM, Phompida S, Jelinek T.Distribution of the two forms of Plasmodium falciparum erythrocyte binding antigen-175 (eba-175) gene in Lao PDR. *Malar J.* 2003;2:23.
[28] Than AM, Harano T, Harano K, Myint AA, Ogino T, Okadaa S. High incidence of 3-thalassemia, hemoglobin E, and glucose-6-phosphate dehydrogenase deficiency in populations of malaria-endemic southern Shan State, Myanmar. *Int J Hematol.* 2005;82:119-23.

[29] Win N, Lwin AA, Oo MM, Aye KS, Soe S, Okada S. Hemoglobin E prevalence in malaria-endemic villages in Myanmar. *Acta Med Okayama*. 2005;59:63-6.

[30] Zhou SS, Tang LH, Sheng HF, Wang Y. Malaria situation in the People' s Republic of China in 2004. *Zhongguo Ji Sheng Chong Xue Yu Ji Sheng Chong Bing Za Zhi.* 2006;24:1-3.

[31] Sheng HF, Zhou SS, Gu ZC, Zheng X. Malaria situation in the People's Republic of China in 2002. *Zhongguo Ji Sheng Chong Xue Yu Ji Sheng Chong Bing Za Zhi.* 2003;21:193-6.

[32] Zhu HM, Li J, Zheng H.Human natural infection of Plasmodium knowlesi. *Zhongguo Ji Sheng Chong Xue Yu Ji Sheng Chong Bing Za Zhi*. 2006;24:70-1.

[33] Singh TG, Singh RK, Singh EY. A study of knowledge about malaria and treatment seeking behaviour in two tribal communities of Manipur. *Indian J Public Health.* 2003;47:61-5.

Chapter 3

ALTERATION IN BASIC LABORATORY RESULTS IN MALARIA: A SUMMARY FROM THAI CASES

ABSTRACT

Malaria is a common febrile illness in the tropics including Thailand. Similar to other blood infections, the alteration in basic laboratory results in the patients infected with malaria. The changes in complete blood count, urinalysis as well as basic clinical chemistry parameter in malaria are mentioned. In this article, the author will summarize the basic findings on basic laboratory results. Also, the summary of such findings from Thai cases in the previous reports will be performed.

LABORATORY PRESENTATION IN MALARIA

Malaria is a common febrile illness in the tropics including Thailand. Similar to other blood infections, the alteration in basic laboratory results in the patients infected with malaria.

Concerning the laboratory abnormality in malaria, aberration of hematological laboratory parameters is common. Presentation of inclusions as malarial parasite or malarial pigment is the key for diagnosis of malarial infection. Concerning the three series of blood cells, all are affected by malarial infection. Considering red blood cell, anemia, as a resulted from malarial infection, is widely mentioned. Severe and refractory anemia leading to hypoxia and cardiac decompensation in malarial patients [1]. Those fatal malaria are common for falciparum malaria. Several mechanisms have been proposed to play a role in the pathogenesis of malarial anemia, such as erythrocyte lysis and phagocytosis, and sequestration of parasitized red blood cells [1]. Concerning erythrocyte lysis, it is believed to due to several cytokine productions especially TNF [2]. Waitumbi *et al* looked for changes in the red cell surfaces of children with severe malarial anemia that could explain this accelerated destruction and they found that red cells from patients with severe anemia were more susceptible to phagocytosis and also showed increased surface IgG and deficiencies in CR1 and CD55 compared with controls [3]. In addition, red cell surface CD59 was elevated in cases of severe anemia compared with asymptomatic controls but not as compared with symptomatic controls [3]. Waitumbi *et al* concluded that the surface of red cells of children with severe *Plasmodium falciparum* anemia was modified by the deposition of IgG and alterations in the levels of complement regulatory proteins and these changes could contribute to the accelerated destruction of red cells in these patients by mechanisms such as phagocytosis or complement-mediated lysis [3]. Concerning microvascular sequestration of parasitized red blood cells, Weatherall *et al* said that after an acute malarial infection there was a steady fall in the haemoglobin level with an inappropriate reticulocyte response [4]. They proposed that this form of anemia might result from a combination of acute sequestration of iron in the reticuloendothelial system associated with a shortened red cell survival [4]. In addition, Davis *et al* studied the mathmetical model of the microvascular sequestation phenomenon and found the mean fall in hematocrit over 84 hours in the patients conformed to a three-term equation [5]. Concerning the autoimmune hemolytic anemia, this phenomenon is very rare in malaria and not proposed as a common mechanism for malarial anemia [1].

In additional to hematological manifestation, the other uncommon clinical presentations of malaria are also documented. Hepatic manifestation is an interesting uncommon presentation of malaria. The abnormality of liver function test is also reported. Recently, Wiwanitkit proposed that jaundice is not an uncommon presentation in the patients with malarial infection [6]. Yuda and Ishino said that malarial transmission to the human host was established by sporozoite infection of the liver and sporozoites are released from the mosquito salivary glands and carried by the blood flow to the liver sinusoid [7]. They noted that traversal of the sinusoidal cell layer and subsequent hepatocyte infection were the most important events in sporozoite liver invasion, but the molecular basis of both events remained to be elucidated [7]. They also said that this process was homologous to midgut epithelium penetration by the malarial ookinete, because identical or paralogous genes were critically involved in both processes [7]. Recent studies had revealed that NKT cells participate in some types of liver injuries especially for malaria hepatitis [8]. Malarial cirrhosis is an interesting topic of malarial infection. In 1981, Islam *et al* performed a clinical analysis of 293 cases of cirrhosis from two moderate-sized hospitals in Dacca and found that 10.24 % of the patients had the past history of malaria [9]. Until present, it can be confirmed that there is malarial hepatitis but the existence of malarial cirrhosis is controversy [10 – 12]. However, Rothenberg *et al* stated that chronic liver diseases, especially cirrhosis, were not known as ascertained late lesions of malaria [13].

Alteration in Basic Laboratory Results in Malaria

As previously mentioned, the changes in complete blood count, urinalysis as well as basic clinical chemistry parameter in malaria can be seen. The summary of such important findings from Thai cases in the previous reports will be performed.

Anemia in Malaria

There are many literatures on malarial anemia in Thailand. Forty years ago, Panikbutr et al studied anemia in malaria in relation to the species of parasites and some clinical aspects [14].

The results are as follows:- 1. 94.7 per cent of their case series had anemia during infection, from which 61.4 per cent, 32.0 per cnet and 1.3 per cent were mild, moderate and severe anemic respectively. 2 [14]. From the series, the close relationship between degree of anemia, chronicity of the disease and age of the patients were demonstrated and the correlation between species of parasites and degree of anemia in chronic group were also demonstrated whereas in acute group this relation was not found [14]. Of interest, the correlation between intensity of parasites and degree of anemia could not be demonstrated in this study [14]. Recently, Yamokgul et al compared of anemia in patients with falciparum malaria in endemic area before and after radical treatment [15]. Comparison was done by measuring of their hematocrit values five times on day 0, 14, 28, 42 and 56 [15]. The study found that, the anemia proportion of falciparum patient significant differed from vivax patients and non-malaria cases [15]. The anemia of falciparum patient was not depended on parasitemia levels and the rehabililation of the anemia was depended on the duration after received radical treatment [15]. In addition, the anemia of falciparum patients resisted to antimalarial drug was significant higher than the patients responded [15]. From this study, the anemia of these patients was mostly chronic state, which could be anticipated that it depended on three factors, re-infections, malnutrition and antimalarial drug resistance [15].

Of interest, malarial anemia in Thai patients should be carefully differentially diagnosed from the other common underlying endemic hematological problems including thalassmeia and hemoglobinopathy. Indeed, both thalassmeia and hemoglobinopathy are common in Thailand and believed to be the result of natural selection process to the previous high density of malaria in Southeast Asia.

Abnormal of Liver Function Test in Malaria

Abnormal of liver function test in malaria has been continuously reported in Thai malarial patients. More than 40 years, the impaired liver function test was firstly documented as an important laboratory manifestation in Thai patients infected with malaria [16]. Recently, Wilairatana et al studied liver involvement in cerebral malaria [17].In this work, elevated levels of aspartate aminotransferase (AST), alanine aminotransferase (ALT), bilirubin, alkaline phosphatase, and prothrombin time were observed in 92.2%, 54.7%, 92.2%, 7.8%, and 0 % of the patients, respectively [17]. In addition, liver profile values did not differ significantly between the survivors and non-survivors, but other indicators of severity such as coma score, renal function, and acidbase balance were significantly more deranged in non-survivors [17]. They concluded that falciparum malaria was associated with hepatic abnormalities but that fatal outcomes might be attributed to physiologic abnormalities other than liver dysfunction [17].

Abnormal of Urinalysis in Malaria

The effect of malaria on kidney is not common and it is hardly to see abnormal of urinalysis as manifestation of malaria. However, the renal complication of malaria can be seen and the abnormal of urinalysis can be detected in these cases. In summary, renal ischmia in malaria can therefore be induced by a combination of several pathophysiological changes

[18]. These changes include hypovolemia, hyperviscosity and catecholamine release. Renal ischemia may be of great enough degree to cause renal failure [18]. Acute tubular necrosis, the principal pathologic lesion in falciparum malaria-induced ARF, is mediated by a complex interaction of mechanical, immunologic, cytokine, humoral, acute phase response, non specific factors, and hemodynamics factors [19]. Parasitized erythrocytes express a central role in all aforementioned pathogenic factors of acute renal failure [19].

Electrolyte Disturbance in Malaria

Electrolyte disturbance can be seen in malaria. Of the four major electrolytes, sodium, potassium, chloride and bicarbornate, the disturbance of potassemia is the most important disturbance leading to several clinical implications. However, there are limited studies on this area in Thailand. Here, the author performed a retrospective study to find whether there was correlation between the serum potassium and some clinical parameters of the patients with falciparum malaria. Ninty-three patients with falciparum were included into this study. At present, these 39 cases had a mean (SD) age of 29.78 (17.27) (range = 1 – 82 years). Average duration of present illness was 6.61 $\pm$ 4.94 days. On admission, the average serum potassium was 3.80 $\pm$ 0.47 mg/dL (range, 3.3 to 4.7 mg/dL). Concerning the multiple logistic regression analysis, no significant correlation was found between serum potassium level and the other parameters. According to this study, the author found no significant correlation between the serum potassium level and the studied patients' characteristics I(age, sex, duration of present illness, duration of hospitalization, white blood count, hematocrit and platelet count) as well. In conclusion, the author could not demonstrate the correlation between the serum potassium level and those studied parameters among the subjects.

References

[1] McDevitt MA, Xie J, Gordeuk V, Bucala R. The anemia of malaria infection: role of inflammatory cytokines. *Curr Hematol Rep* 2004;3:97-106.

[2] McGuire W, Knight JC, Hill AV, Allsopp CE, Greenwood BM, Kwiatkowski D. Severe malarial anemia and cerebral malaria are associated with different tumor necrosis factor promoter alleles. *J Infect Dis* 1999;179:287-90.

[3] Waitumbi JN, Opollo MO, Muga RO, Misore AO, Stoute JA. Red cell surface changes and erythrophagocytosis in children with severe plasmodium falciparum anemia. *Blood* 2000;95:1481-6.

[4] Weatherall DJ, Abdalla S, Pippard MJ. The anemia of Plasmodium falciparum malaria. *Ciba Found Symp* 1983;94:74-97.

[5] Davis TM, Krishna S, Looareesuwan S, Supanaranond W, Pukrittayakamee S, Attatamsoonthorn K, White NJ. Erythrocyte sequestration and anemia in severe falciparum malaria. Analysis of acute changes in venous hematocrit using a simple mathematical model. *J Clin Invest* 1990;86:793-800.

[6] Wiwanitkit V. Jaundice as co-presentation in Thai malarial patients. *J Indian Med Assoc.* 2004 Feb;102(2):107.

[7] Yuda M, Ishino T. Liver invasion by malarial parasites--how do malarial parasites break through the host barrier? *Cell Microbiol.* 2004 Dec;6(12):1119-25.

[8] Tsutsui H, Adachi K, Seki E, Nakanishi K. Cytokine-induced inflammatory liver injuries. *Curr Mol Med.* 2003 Sep;3(6):545-59.

[9] Islam N, Khan M, Ahmed Z. Cirrhosis of liver. *Bangladesh Med Res Counc Bull* 1981;7:45-51.

[10] Mahi PN, Tandon HD. Malarial hepatitis. J Indiana State Med Assoc 1955;25:507-11.

[11] Gyergyay F, Hermann E. Etiopathogenetic factors in liver cirrhosis. *Med Interna* (Bucur) 1956;8:669-79.

[12] Franken HF, Snoos A. Is there a malaria cirrhosis? *Munch Med Wochenschr* 1966; 108:879-83.

[13] Rothenberg G, Schubert S. Assessment of late complications of malaria in travelers to the tropics. *Z Gesamte Inn Med* 1983;38:46-7.

[14] Panikbutr N, Jeumtrakul P, Srichaikul T. Anemia in malaria in relation to the species of parasites and some clinical aspects. *J Med Assoc Thai* 1966; 49(4): 281-291.

[15] Yamokgul P, Bualombai P, Srisuwannathat V, Buafuengklin A, Tapingkae M. Comparison of anemia in patients with falciparum malaria in endemic area before and after radical treatment. *J Health Sci* 1995; 4(4): 304-311.

[16] Techakrasaya C, Jinayhon S, Pamornsatit S. The study of liver function tests and paper electrophoresis of the protein in malarial disease. 1962; 9(2): 10-14.

[17] Wilairatana P, Pongponrat E, Riganti M, Vannaphan S, Looareesuwan S. Liver involvement in cerebral malaria . *Mahidol Univ J* 1996; 3(1): 11-14.

[18] Sitprija V, Vongsthongsri M, Poshyachinda V, Arthachinta S. Pathogenesis of renal failure in malaria. *J Med Assoc Thai* 1978; 61(Suppl 1): 71-73.

[19] Eiam-ong S. Current knowledge in falciparum malaria-induced acute renal failure. *J Med Assoc Thai* 2002; 85(Suppl 1): S16-S24.

Chapter 4

MALARIAL VECTOR: A SUMMARY ON RESEARCH IN THAILAND

ABSTRACT

Malaria is a vector borne parasitic disease. Here, the details of mosquito vector of malaria and its correlation to the life cycle of malaria will be reviewed and discussed. In addition, a summary on malarial vector research in Thailand will be summarized. A wide range of researches cover vector entomology, vector epidemiology as well as vector control can be found.

INTRODUCTION TO MALARIAL VECTOR

Malaria is a protozoan infection transmitted by the biting female Anopheles mosquito. These mosquitoes bite during the nighttime hours, from dusk to dawn. It cannot be casually transmitted from person to person but it is possible to spread malaria via blood or placenta transfusions [1 – 2]. Symptoms of malaria include fever, shivering, pain and vomiting [3]. Some serious presentation such as generalized convulsions and coma are also documented [1 – 2]. However, some uncommon presentation of malarial infection such as epistaxis and hypermenorrhea are mentioned [3]. In addition, as many as half a billion people worldwide are left with chronic anemia due to malaria infections. The malarial symptoms of the disease usually begin 1 week to 2 weeks after being bit [1 – 2].

According to the World Health Organization, malaria infects between 300 and 500 million people every year in Africa, South Asia, Southeast Asia, the Middle East, Oceania, and Central and South America. The disease affects approximately 40% of the world's population and over one million of the infected die each year [4]. The corresponding pathogen is *Plasmodium* spp. It is the most well known mosquito-borne disease. For several centuries, this disease has been documented as an important threatens to humans. In addition, it is important problem for farm animals especially chicken. There is also a specific museum for malaria. In the Museum for the History of the Pavia University, Italy, important materials on the role of this scientist in the history of malariology are kept [5]. Malaria is accepted as one of the most important tropical infectious disease. However, the spread of malaria to the non-tropical countries has been mentioned for years.

The mosquito vector is *Anopheles* spp. Like all other mosquitoes, the anophelines breed in water, and each species having its preferred breeding grounds, feeding patterns and resting place [6]. Their sensitivity to insecticides is also highly variable [6]. Concerning the life cycle, Plasmodium develops in the gut of the mosquito and is passed on in the saliva of an infected insect each time it takes a new blood meal [6] (Figure 1). The parasites are then carried by the blood in the victim's liver where they invade the cells and multiply [6] (Table 1). After 9-16 days they return to the blood and penetrate the red cells, where they multiply again, progressively breaking down the red cells [6].

Table 1 Number of merozoite of pre-erythrocyte and erythrocyte stages of different malaria species.

Type of Malaria	Number of Merozoite	
	Pre-erythrocyte stage	Erythrocyte Stage
Vivax	10,000	12
Falciparum	30,000	16
Ovale	15,000	8
Malaria	15,000	8

The bioecological parameters, which were of special importance in the epidemiology of malaria, include three levels: the nature of mosquito-man contacts, the susceptibility of the mosquito to the pathogen and multiplication of the latter, and the transmission. Hurd and Carter suggested that programmed cell death occurred during the early stages of the development of the malaria parasite in its vector [7]. Hurd and Carter noted that malaria infection induced apoptosis in the cells of two mosquito tissues, the midgut and the follicular epithelium [7]. They noted that putative signal molecules that might induce parasite and vector apoptosis included nitric oxide, reactive nitrogen intermediates, oxygen radicals and endocrine balance [7]. Finally, They concluded that programmed cell death might play a critical role in regulation of infection by the parasite and the host, and contributed to the success or not of parasite establishment and host survival.

The bioecological parameters, which were of special importance in the epidemiology of malaria, include three levels: the nature of mosquito-man contacts, the susceptibility of the mosquito to the pathogen and multiplication of the latter, and the transmission. Hurd and Carter suggested that programmed cell death occurred during the early stages of the development of the malaria parasite in its vector [8]. Hurd and Carter noted that malaria infection induced apoptosis in the cells of two mosquito tissues, the midgut and the follicular epithelium [8]. They noted that putative signal molecules that might induce parasite and vector apoptosis included nitric oxide, reactive nitrogen intermediates, oxygen radicals and endocrine balance [8]. Finally, They concluded that programmed cell death might play a critical role in regulation of infection by the parasite and the host, and contributed to the success or not of parasite establishment and host survival.

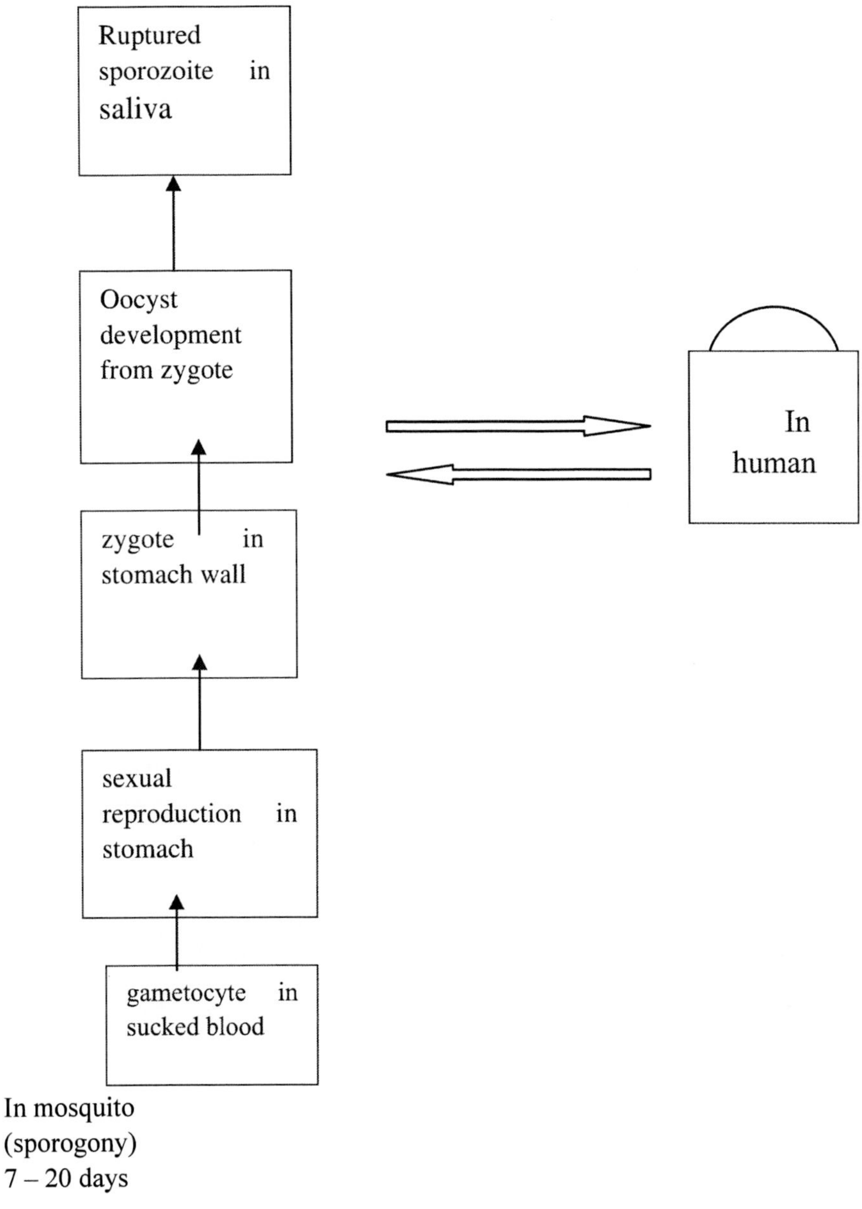

Figure 1. Life cycle of malaria.

ANOPHELES MOSQUITO, VECTOR OF MALARIA

Anopheles is a genus of mosquito causing several tropical mosquito-borne diseases especially for malaria. Among the insects that serve as vectors for parasitic diseases, this genus is arguably the most important [9]. Of the approximately 400 species of *Anopheles*, about two dozen serve as vectors for malaria (*Plasmodium* spp.in humans and the mosquitoes also serve as the vector for canine heart worm.(*Dirofilaria immitis*) [9]. Several species of

Anopheline mosquitoes can be the vectors of malaria. In 2004, Ool *et al* performed a study to examine the species of anopheline mosquitoes in Myanmar and found that out of 36 species of anophelines distributed throughout the country, 10 species were found to be infected with the malaria parasite [10]. Gunasekaran *et al* performed a similar study in Koraput district of Orissa, India, which is highly malarious [11]. According to their study, a total of 62,086 anophelines belonging to 22 species and two varieties were collected, including 8 species of anophelines which are recognized malarial vectors in India [11]. In this study, a total of 24154 mosquitoes were dissected and 18 mosquitoes belonging to four species, *Anopheles fluviatilis*, *Anopheles annularis*, *Anopheles culicifacies* and *Anopheles aconitus* were found with the gut/gland infection [11].

Norris said that human malaria was truly a disease of global proportions and was one of the most broadly distributed vector-borne infections and Anopheline mosquitoes were the exclusive vectors of human malaria [12]. Norris noted that a handful of species predominated as the most notorious malaria vectors, but the species and forms involved in the transmission of human malaria world-wide were incredibly diverse [12]. Norris proposed that many of the anophelines that vector malaria existed as members of species complexes that often contain vector and non-vector species and single anopheline species often exhibit significant heterogeneity across the species' range [12]. Norris said that this phenotypic and genotypic plasticity exacerbated the difficulties in identification of vector populations and implementation of effective surveillance and control strategies [12]. Norris mentioned that polytene chromosome investigations were among the first to provide researchers with tangible genetic markers that could be used to differentiate between what were recognised as species and chromosomal forms of anopheline mosquitoes [12]. Norris concluded that many new molecular markers had proven useful in a wide variety of applications including molecular taxonomy, evolutionary systematics, population genetics, genetic mapping, and investigation of defined phenotypes [12].

Summary on Malarial Vector Research in Thailand

Thailand is a country in tropical Asia with the high prevalence of malaria. There are several previous researches on malarial vector in Thailand. A wide range of researches cover vector entomology, vector epidemiology as well as vector control can be found.

Vector Entomology

Historically, *Anophles leucosphyrus* is the main mosquito contributing the malaria from monkey to human, human to human and human to monkey in the early era [13]. This vector lived in the rain forest and passed the process of evolution into many problematic species at present. In Thailand, *Anopheles dirus* is the most problematic species [13]. This species is the problematic species with high rate of drug resistance and widely distributed in Thailand and Myanmar [14]. This species are common in a forest wood-extraction area, an irrigated plain area near foothills, a coastal plain near the foothill area, as well as a hilly area [14]. Three subgroups can be divided due to the habitats: form D in the dark forests, form A in the junctions between hill and coastal plain and form C in forest of lime mountain [13]. For the other species, *Anopheles minimus*, *Anopheles maculatus* (form A) or *Anopheles pseudowillmori* are also proposed as occasional vector for malaria in Thailand [13].

Recently, Sucharit and Komalamisra performed a study aiming at differentiation of anopheles minimus species complex by RAPD-PCR technique [15]. In this work, amplification of random regions of genomic DNA using 10-base primers in the random-amplified polymorphic DNA polymerase chain reaction (RAPD-PCR) was used to differentiate *Anopheles minimus* A and *Anopheles minimus* C [15]. They concluded that *Anopheles minimus* species A and C can be differentiated by RAPD-PCR technique [15]. According to another study by Koottathep et al, enzyme-linked immunosorbent assay (ELISA) was used to detect the circumsporozoite (CS) proteins of *Plasmodium falciparum* and *Plasmodium vivax* sporozoites in 18 Anopheles species collected from human and buffalo in a forest-fringe area of Northwest Thailand [16]. Of interest, in non-vector mosquitoes; Pf CS protein was detected in *Anopheles* maculatus, *Anopheles vagus* and *Anopheles hyrcanus* gr; *Plasmodium vivax* CS protein was detected in *Anopheles annularis*, *Anopheles maculatus*, *Anopheles* nivipes, *Anopheles.hyrcanus* gr. and *Anopheles culicifacies* [16]. Therefore, these mosquitoes should be considered as potential vectors of malaria, but their vector status requires confirmation [16].

Vector Epidemiology

There are several studies on the vector epidemiology in Thailand. For example, Yantaksa and Suwonkerd performed an interesting study on unusual breeding places of Anopheles minimus This study was carried out in a rural village of Chun District, Payao Province, Northern Thailand [17]. The study area was plain and paddy field which was not usual breeding place for this anopheles [17]. According to this study, the Anopheles minimus larvae were found in 6.25 per cent of the larval survey (5 out of 8) and the adult mosquitoes were found in 14.3 per cent of the mosquito collection (1 out of 7) [17]. This study confirmed the presence of *Anopheles minimus* in unfavorable conditions in Northern Thailand [17]. Marrat and Veerakul performed another study to determine seasonal variation of anopheline mosquitoes at Pakmoon Dam Project and its adjacent areas, Ubon-Rachathani province in Northeastern Region of Thailand [18]. The result of the study indicated that the population density of each collected species of anopheline mosquitoes varied widely throughout the year and each species had its own population density pattern which may indicate that it could have been due to the competition among the anopheline species and with other blood-feeding insects [18]. In addition, the result of comparison of 3 collecting methods used for adult anopheline mosquitoes collection during investigation showed that light trapping method yielded the best results [18]. Another short report on the study of malaria mosquito from Mae Jam districtin Northern Thailand was performed by Wiwanitkit and Suyaphan during summer 2001 [19]. In this study, the null prevalence of malaria mosquito and larvae was observed [19]. This finding is according to the nature of the community as closed community and corresponding to the null prevalence of malaria blood survey in the same period [19]. In addition, Wiwanitkit also reported a significant correlation between prevalence of malaria and altitude [20]. This implies the limitation of vector distribution to the high altitude [20].

Vector Control

There are also many studies on the malarial vector control in Thailand. In order to get success in prevention and control of mosquito-borne disease, updating on the data of those diseases are necessary. Basic information is required before planning and launching of any preventive strategies. New technology should be applied for this purpose. Vector control is a basic useful primary prevention that can be applied for all mosquito-borne diseases. Since all mosquito-borne diseases are vector-borne diseases, therefore, the control of vector is rational in prevention. Historically, Mulla said that control technology in the first half of the 20th century was relatively simple, utilizing source reduction, larvivorous fish, petroleum hydrocarbon oils, and some simple synthetic and botanical materials and during the 2nd half of the 20th century, however, various classes of synthetic organic chemicals, improved petroleum oil formulations, insect growth regulators, synthetic pyrethroids, and microbial control agents were developed and employed in mosquito control and control of other disease-vectoring insects [21]. These methods are also launched and tested in Thailand.

Most of the studies on vector control in Thailand focus on the use of insecticide. Recently, Pukpibul et al evaluatedof a comparative field trial of DDT, Deltamethrin and Lambdacyhalothrin as residual sprays for malaria control in difference endemic areas of Thailand, Tak, Surat Thani, Chumphon, Kanchanaburi and Chanthaburi [22]. The methods used in these study were both entomological and epidemiological procedures including the detection of malaria cases in the study areas [22]. In this study, lambdacyhalothrin and DDT spray had reduced the densities as well as parous rates of malaria vector *Anopheles minimus* [22]. These findings were not observed in the areas with deltamethrin sprays. Susceptibility tests showed that the malaria vector *Anopheles minimus* was highly susceptible to these three insecticides. DDT had prolonged residual effect of six months on hard wood surface, followed by lambdacyhalothrin (4 months) and deltamethrin (3 months) [22]. Significant reduction of annual parasite incidence was observed with lambdacyhalothrin while the incidence was found to increase with deltamethrin and DDT [22]. There was also no difference in the acceptability and immediate toxicity of deltamethrin and lambdacyhalothrin [22]. Another field trial using lambdacyhalothrin as residual spray at a target dosage of 30 mg./m exponent 2 was carried out to determine the efficacy of insecticide on malaria vectors and its impact in controlling malaria under field conditions [23]. In this work, surface bioassay test results gave 100 per cent mortality of *Anopheles dirus* after one year of single application of lambdacyhalothin 30mg./m exponent 2 on hard wood surface [23]. Mortality of *Anopheles minimus* collected from window trap was decreased to 60 per cent after 3 months of insecticide application [23].

The combination between bed net and insecticide is also widely tried in Thailand. Practically, mosquito net impregnated with permethrin at dosage 0.2 gm/m exponent 2 on mosquitonets made of cotton, nylon and polyester which are usually used by villagers entomoligical team [24]. In a recent interesting study, field WHO Bioassay tests to determine residual effects of permethrin treated mosquito net were conducted in Chumphon province [24]. Using 70 per cent mortality as criteria residual effects of permethrin at 0.2 gm/m exponent 2 were 6, 5 and 3 months on polyester, Cotton and nylon respectively [24]. It was also observe that the knock down effects of permethrin were high within 3 months after impregnation [24].

However, another study documented that the human biting rate of mosquito in the house using and not using permethrin treated bed net was not significant different [25].

REFERENCES

[1] Vector borne diseases. Available at http://www.fpnotebook.com/ID211.htm

[2] Changes in the Incidence of Vector-Borne Diseases Attributable to Climate Change. Available at http://www.ciesin.org/TG/HH/veclev2.html

[3] Suyaphun A, Wiwanitkit V, Suwansaksri J, Nithiuthai S, Sritar S, Suksirisampant W, Fongsungnern A. Malaria among hilltribe communities in northern Thailand: a review of clinical manifestations. Southeast. *Asian J Trop Med Public Health*. 2002; 33 Suppl 3: 14-5.

[4] Schlagenhauf P. Malaria: from prehistory to present. *Infect. Dis Clin North Am.* 2004; 18: 189-205.

[5] Mazzarello P, Calligaro AL. Golgi's documents about the history of malaria. *Med Secoli*. 1998; 10: 495-510.

[6] Malaria. Available at http://www-micro.msb.le.ac.uk/224/Malaria.html

[7] Hurd H, Carter V. The role of programmed cell death in Plasmodium-mosquito interactions. *Int J Parasitol*. 2004; 34: 1459-72.

[8] Hurd H, Carter V. The role of programmed cell death in Plasmodium-mosquito interactions. *Int J Parasitol*. 2004; 34: 1459-72.

[9] Anopheles spp. Available at

[10] http://www.biosci.ohio- state.edu/~parasite/anopheles.html

[11] Ool TT, Storch V, Becker N. Review of the anopheline mosquitoes of Myanmar. *J Vector Ecol*. 2004; 29:21-40.

[12] Gunasekaran K, Sahu SS, Parida SK, Sadanandane C, Jambulingam P, Das PK. Anopheline fauna of Koraput district, Orissa state, with particular reference to transmission of malaria. *Indian J Med Res*. 1989; 89: 340-3.

[13] Norris DE. Genetic markers for study of the anopheline vectors of human malaria. *Int J Parasitol*. 2002; 32: 1607-15.

[14] Baimai V. Evolution of anopheles, vector of malaria. *Warasan Malaria* 1994; 29: 68.

[15] Oo TT, Storch V, Becker N. Anopheles dirus and its role in malaria transmission in Myanmar. *J Vector. Ecol*. 2003; 28: 175-83.

[16] Sucharit S, Komalamisra N. Differentiation of anopheles minimus species complex by RAPD-PCR technique. *J Med Assoc Thai*. 1998; 80: 598-602.

[17] Koottathep S, Somboon P, Khamboonruang C. Detection of circumsporozoite proteins in Anopheles mosquitoes in a forest-fringe area of Northwest Thailand by ELISA. *Chiang Mai Med Bull* 1993; 32(1): 9-12

[18] Yantaksa P, Suwonkerd W. Study on unusual breeding places of Anopheles minimus (theobald) in Payao Province. *Commun Dis J.* 1994; 20(3): 195-201.

[19] Marrat T, Veerakul S. Seasonal variation of anopheline mosquitoes at Pakmoon Dam Project and its adjacent areas, Ubon-Rachathani, Thailand. *J Health Sci* 1996; 5(1): 118-124.

[20] Wiwanitkit V, Suyaphan A. The survey of malarial mosquito of Mae Suk subdistrict, Mae Jam, Chiangmai Province : a short report. *Lampang Hosp Bull* 2003 ; 24(1): 56-58.

[21] Wiwanitkit V. Correlation between prevalence of malaria and altitude, a study in a rural endemic area of Thailand. *Haema*. 2006; 9(1): 56-58.

[22] Mulla MS. Mosquito control then, now, and in the future. *J Am Mosq Control Assoc*. 1994; 10:574-84.

[23] Pukpibul A, Sudathip P, Guntasri T. Evaluation of a comparative field trial of DDT, Deltamethrin and Lambdacyhalothrin as residual sprays for malaria control. *Commun Dis J*. 1998; 24(1): 93-99.

[24] Nutsathapana S, Pukpibul A, Mongklangkul P. Field trial of the insecticide lambdacyhalothrin as residual spray for malaria control in Thailand. *Commun Dis J* 1997; 23(3): 369-376.

[25] Temahivong T, Boonyang J, Saeoue W, Jaisawang C. Residual effect of permethrin impregnated mosquito net using anopheles minimus theobald (diptera : culicidae). *Commun Dis J* 1993; 19: 195-200.

[26] Sae-ui V, Suttirattananimit T, Kongkaew S, Boonyung S. A study on the efficacy of permethrin-treated bed net in control of mosquitoes. *Warasan Malaria* 1994; 29(2): 60-66.

Chapter 5

NATURAL SELECTION OF MALARIA IN THAILAND

ABSTRACT

The high prevalence of malaria in Southeast Asia including Thailand is believed to be a big hazard to the population in this area. This problem has been exist here for thousand years. Adaptation of the population in this area following the principle of natural selection can be expected. The good examples for natural selection of malaria in Thailand are the co-existence of high prevalence of thalassemia as well as glucose-6-phosphate dehydrogenase deficiency.

INTRODUCTION TO MALARIA IN SOUTHEAST ASIA

Tropical Asia is the well-known endemic area of malaria. In Southeast Asia, the high prevalence of malaria is mentioned. Hay *et al* noted that stratifying the malaria extent by endemically class and examining regional differences highlighted that nearly 1 billion people are exposed to hypoendemic and mesoendemic malaria in southeast Asia [1]. In Thailand, noted that rubber tapers in southern region had the highest malaria incidence rate (46.29%) [2]. Similar high prevalence among the hill tribes in the northern region is also noted [3]. Of interest, Wiwanitkit recently reported for the impact of migration of the populations from Myanmar to Thailand on the prevalence of malaria in a Thai-Myanmar border area namely Bangsaparn [4]. Chaveepojnkamjorn and Pichainarong also reported a similar finding in another Thai-Myanmar border area namely [5]. They noted that *Plasmodium falciparum* was the major type of the malaria (60.8%) [5]. A cross-sectional survey of the malaria prevalence among mobile Cambodians in Aranyaprathet, at the Thai-Cambodia border, was conducted in November 2000 [6]. According to this study, the overall prevalence rate was 2.4%, with 93.75% of the infections being due to Plasmodium vivax and 6.25% due to *Plasmodium falciparum* [6]. Kitvatanachai *et al* said that factors associated with malaria infection included being male, being in the 10-59 year age group, having a lower level of education and frequent trans-border crossing [6].

In other Indochina countries, the high prevalence of malaria is noted. Singhasivanon said that there was great diversity in disease patterns in the Indochina countries and at subnational administrative unit area level in each country, so that in the region as a whole there was marked asymmetry in disease distribution, with many areas of high endemicity [7]. Singhasivanon noted that focal expansion of maps in the vicinity of international border areas delineated the differential trans-border malaria distribution that presented a challenge for disease control [7]. Singhasivanon also noted that the malaria pattern was also depicted in environmental context against regional elevation and forest cover profiles, which affected mosquito breeding site distribution and agricultural activity [7]. Concerning Cambodia, Denis and Meek noted that there were around half a million cases of malaria with 5-10,000 deaths per year [8]. They said that malaria control was hampered In Cambodia by multiple drug resistance of *Plasmodium falciparum*, inaccessibility to the major vector, poor security in most malarious areas, and lack of resources [8]. Concerning Laos, Pholsena said that malaria was endemic in all 17 provinces of Laos and transmission was perennial with a "seasonal peak" coinciding with the rainy season [9]. Pholsena noted that the vectors *Anopheles minimus* and *Anopheles balabacensis* in Laos remained susceptible to insecticide and multidrug resistance was not a problem [9]. Concerning Vietnam, malaria is still the most common infectious cause of mortality and morbidity in Vietnam as it is in many developing countries in the tropic [10]. These reports can confirm the importance and high prevalence of malaria in Thailand and nearby countries.

Natural Selection: What is It?

Natural selection is an important way of evolution process. It is the process by which individual organisms with favorable traits are more likely to survive and reproduce [11]. Natural selection works on the whole individual, but only the heritable component of a trait will be passed on to the offspring, with the result that favorable, heritable traits become more common in the next generation [11]. Given enough time, this passive process can result in adaptations and speciation [11]. Evolution of the human genome under selective pressure from malaria is a good example of natural selection [12]. It is difficult to overestimate the evolutionary pressures exerted over the past few thousand years by endemic malaria [13]. For many human populations, endemic malaria became an evolutionary emergency. In such pressing circumstances, genetic traits which ordinarily would carry with them an intolerable genetic load actually increase in frequency [13]. Thus, although a few antimalarial red cell characteristics such as Duffy negativity are evidently innocuous, the majority of malaria-selected traits are not [13]. Ovalocytosis, the abnormal hemoglobins and G-6-PD deficiencies are all quite deleterious in the homo- or hemizygote [13].

Of several disorders, the most well-known is sickle cell disorder [14]. Usually in a population the frequency of lethal recessive genes decreases by eliminating the homozygous individuals. In sickle cell disease the decrease of the frequency of mutant recessive genes does not take place [14]. The fact that a gene which in the homozygous state expressed a serious clinical picture reaches a high frequency in a population can be explained only by a process of natural selection that would offer the heterozygous an advantage [14]. It is accepted that sickle cell disorder is the good model for natural selection in medicine. This disorder is believed to be a result of natural selection process to response to the high prevalence of malaria in African ancestors. However, in addition to natural selection on human genome, the natural selection on malarial genome also leads to the problem of drug resistance malaria at present [15].

NATURAL SELECTION OF MALARIA IN THAILAND

The natural selection process of malaria in Thailand is also documented. Similar to the correlation between sickle cell disorder and malaria in Africa. Several hematological abnormalities in Thailand are mentioned for its correlation to the natural selection process of malaria. The good examples for natural_selection of malaria in Thailand are the co-existence of high prevalence of thalassemia as well as glucose-6-phosphate dehydrogenase deficiency.

A. Hemoglobin E Disroder

A well-known hemoglobinopathy, hemoglobin E is peak endemic in this area, in northeastern of Thailand and Laos [16 - 17]. Due to the recent study of Dode et al, high prevalence of Hb E and alpha-thalassaemia were found among the Southeast Asian refugees [18]. However, there are some other hemoglobinopathies, such as Hb Tak, Hb Suandok, Hb Mahidol, in Southeast Asia as well. Heterozygotes and homozygotes for HbE (beta 26, GAG-AAG, Glu-Lys) are microcytic, minimally anemic, and asymptomatic [19]. Hemoglobin E has the same electrophoretic mobility on alkaline cellulose acetate as hemoglobin A2 and hemoglobin C, however, the mobility of these hemoglobins differs on agar gel electrophoresis (pH 6.2) and they can be distinguished by this method. The synthesis of hemoglobin E in reticulocytes of A/E heterozygotes and E/E homozygotes appears to be significantly impaired, seems to be in the production of beta E chains, therefore, the Hb E structural gene may be viewed as a beta-thalassemia-like gene. Rees *et al* said that the microcytosis is attributed to the beta thalassemic nature of the beta E gene, whereas the in vitro instability of HbE does not contribute to the phenotype, however, the compound heterozygote state HbE/beta thalassemia results in a variable, and often severe anemia, with the phenotype ranging from transfusion dependence to a complete lack of symptoms [20]. The question of single or multiple origins for HbE in south-east Asia is unresolved. Recombination events producing alpha + thalassaemia deletions are frequent, whereas alpha 0 thalassaemia is produced by a variety of large deletions, each of which has had a single origin [21]. The evidence favoring natural selection by *P. falciparum* malaria as the primary cause of high frequencies of the thalassaemias throughout the tropics and subtropics is documented [21].

In Thailand, Wasi et al firstly studied HbA2 and Hb E quantities by DEAE-Sephadex chromatography in 89 patients with P. *falciparum* malaria [22]. Wasi concluded that *P. falciparum* malaria did not increase the levels of Ab A 2 and Hb E [22]. Wasi noted that the finding of increased Hb A2 concerns *P. vivax* and still remains very important and should be tested in other parts of the world [22]. This study lead to the conclusion that Hb E disorder might be due to the natural selection of malaria. Of interest, the trend of lower Hb in the malaria presented with unknown status of Hb electrophoresis pattern is documented. Pongyingpis found that the value of platelet count, Hb level which tested by the Median test in both sexes were significantly lower in malarial patients than in non-malarial patients [23].

However, this finding might be due to the underlying inherited anemic disease or the malaria-induced anemia.

B. Glucose-6-Phosphate Dehydrogenase Deficiency.

Glucose-6-phosphate dehydrogenase (G6PD, EC1.1.1.49) is an enzyme expressed in all tissues, where it catalyses the first step in the pentose phosphate pathway [24 – 26]. This first reaction in the pathway leads to the production of pentose phosphates and reducing power in the form of NADPH for reductive biosynthesis and maintenance of the cellular redox state [24 – 26]. The defect of this enzyme namely G6PD deficiency is the most common sex linked inherited enzymatic defect, affecting over 400 million persons worldwide [24 – 26]. This disorder can cause hemolytic anemia [24].The prevalence of G6PD deficiency in the Southeast Asia is high. This region is the endemic area of malaria, therefore, it is no doubt for this finding. In this region, the prevalence of G6PD deficiency has been continuously studied. In 1999, Tanphaichitr performed a study in the Thais and found that the prevalence of G6PD deficiency in Thai males ranged from 3-18% depending upon the geographic region and G6PD "Mahidol" (163 Gly --> Ser) was the most common variant found in the Thai population [27]. A similar study was performed in the Thai neonates by *et al* [28]. They found the prevalence of G6PD deficiency as 22.1% in males and 10.1% in females [28]. However, they proposed that G6PD Viangchan (871G>A), not G6PD Mahidol, was the most common deficiency variant in the Thai population [28].

Data from in vitro studies demonstrate impaired growth of *P. falciparum* parasites in G6PD-deficient erythrocytes [29]. Attempts to confirm that G6PD deficiency is protective in field studies of malaria have yielded conflicting results, but recent results from large case control studies conducted in East and West Africa provide strong evidence that the most common African G6PD deficiency variant, G6PD A-, is associated with a significant reduction in the risk of severe malaria for both G6PD female heterozygotes and male hemizygotes [29]. In Thailand, the high prevalence of G6PD deficiency is believed to be due to the natural selection of malaria.

Forty years ago, Kruatrachue et al indicated that lower parasite count in G6PD deficients children was due to the effect of anemia which would be considered as disadvantage of this abnormal gene in the presence of *P. falciparum* infection when it was compared with normal individuals [30]. However, according to a recent study by Insiripong et al, hemoglobin typing and methehoglobin reduction test were performed on 115 malaria patients and compared with controls and it was found that the number of thalassemia/hemoglobinopathies in the malaria group and in the control group were not significantly different and also occurrence of G6PD deficiency in the malaria group was not different from that of the controls [31]. Insiripong et al concluded that there is no protective effect against malaria in G6PD dificiency [31]. Further verification on the correlation between G^PD deficiency, especially in the molecular level, and malaria in Thailand is still needed.

References

[1] Hay SI, Guerra CA, Tatem AJ, Noor AM, Snow RW. The global distribution and population at risk of malaria: past, present, and future. *Lancet Infect Dis*. 2004; 4: 327-36.

[2] Kondrashin AV. Malaria in the WHO Southeast Asia region. *Indian J Malariol*. 1992; 29: 129-60.

[3] Suyaphun A, Wiwanitkit V, Suwansaksri J, Nithiuthai S, Sritar S, Suksirisampant W, Fongsungnern A. Malaria among hilltribe communities in northern Thailand: a review of clinical manifestations. *Southeast Asian J Trop Med Public Health*. 2202; 33 Suppl 3: 14-5.

[4] Wiwanitkit V. High prevalence of malaria in Myanmar migrant workers in a rural district near the Thailand-Myanmar border. *Scand J Infect Dis*. 2002; 34: 236-7.

[5] Chaveepojnkamjorn W, Pichainarong N. Malaria infection among the migrant population along the Thai-Myanmar border area. *Southeast Asian J Trop Med Public Health*. 2004; 35: 48-52.

[6] Kitvatanachai S, Janyapoon K, Rhongbutsri P, Thap LC. A survey on malaria in mobile Cambodians in Aranyaprathet, Sa Kaeo Province, Thailand. *Southeast Asian J Trop Med Public Health*. 2003; 34: 48-53.

[7] Singhasivanon P. Mekong malaria. Malaria, multi-drug resistance and economic development in the greater Mekong subregion of Southeast Asia. *Southeast Asian J Trop Med Public Health*. 1999; 30 Suppl 4: i-iv.

[8] Denis MB, Meek SR. Malaria in Cambodia. *Southeast Asian J Trop Med Public Health*. 1992; 23 Suppl 4: 23-8.

[9] Pholsena K. The malaria situation and antimalaria program in Laos. *Southeast Asian J Trop Med Public Health*. 1992; 23 Suppl 4: 39-42.

[10] Hien TT, VinhChau NV, Vinh NN, Hung NT, Phung MQ, Toan LM, Mai PP, Dung NT, HoaiTam DT, Arnold K. Management of multiple drug-resistant malaria in Viet Nam. *Ann Acad Med Singapore*. 1997; 26: 659-63.

[11] Natural selection. Available on en.wikipedia.org/wiki/Natural_selection

[12] Miller LH. applications for control. *Parassitologia*. 1999 Sep;41(1-3):77-82

[13] Eaton JW, Wood PA. Antimalarial red cells. *Prog Clin Biol Res*. 1984;165:395-412.

[14] Nascutiu AM. Sickle cell anemia and malaria—interferences. *Bacteriol Virusol Parazitol Epidemiol*. 1997 Jan-Jun;42(1-2):11-4.

[15] Mackinnon MJ, Hastings IM. The evolution of multiple drug resistance in malaria parasites. *Trans R Soc Trop Med Hyg*. 1998 Mar-Apr;92(2):188-95.

[16] Fucharoen S, Wanichagoon G. Thalassemia and abnormal hemoglobin. Int J Hematol 2002;76 Suppl 2:83-9

[17] Johnxis JH. Haemoglobinopathies and their occurrence in South East Asia. *Paediatr Indones* 1975;15:112-9

[18] Fucharoen S, Winichagoon P. Hemoglobinopathies in Southeast Asia. *Hemoglobin* 1987;11:65-88

[19] Dode C, Berth A, Bourdillon F, Mahe C, Labie D, Rochette J. Haemoglobin disorders among Southeast-Asian refugees in France. *Acta Haematol* 1987;78:135-6

[20] Rees DC, Styles L, Vichinsky EP, Clegg JB, Weatherall DJ. The hemoglobin E syndromes. *Ann N Y Acad Sci* 1998;850:334-43.
[21] Hill AV. Molecular epidemiology of the thalassaemias (including haemoglobin E. Baillieres *Clin Haematol.* 1992 Jan;5(1):209-38.
[22] Wasi P, Kruatrachue M, Piankijagum A, Pravatmeung P. Hemoglobins A 2 and E levels in malaria. *J Med Assoc Thai* 1971; 54(8): 559-563.
[23] Pongyingpis O. The study of platelet count, hemoglobin level and atypical lymphocyte between Malarial patients and non-Malarial patients. *J Cent Hosp* 1996; 33(1): 41-60.
[24] Mehta A, Mason PJ, Vulliamy TJ. Glucose-6-phosphate dehydrogenase deficiency. *Baillieres Best Pract Res Clin Haematol* 2000;13:21-38
[25] Kaplan M, Hammerman C. Glucose-6-phosphate dehydrogenase
[26] deficiency: a potential source of severe neonatal hyperbilirubinaemia and
[27] kernicterus. *Semin Neonatol* 2002;7:121-8
[28] 26. Evdokimova AI, Ryneiskaia VA, Plakhuta TG. Hemostatic changes in
[29] hereditary hemolytic anemias in children. *Pediatriia.* 1979;8:17-21.
[30] Tanphaichitr VS. Glucose-6-phosphate dehydrogenase deficiency in Thailand; its significance in the newborn. *Southeast Asian J Trop Med Public Health* 1999;30 Suppl 2:75-8
[31] Nuchprayoon I, Sanpavat S, Nuchprayoon S. Glucose-6-phosphate dehydrogenase (G6PD) mutations in Thailand: G6PD Viangchan (871G>A) is the most common deficiency variant in the Thai population. *Hum Mutat* 2002;19:185.
[32] Ruwende C, Hill A. Glucose-6-phosphate dehydrogenase deficiency and malaria. *J Mol Med.* 1998 Jul;76(8):581-8.
[33] Kruatrachue M, Klongkamnuankarn K, Harinasuta C. G-6-PD deficiency and Malaria in Thailand. *J Med Assoc Thai* 1966; 49(12): 945
[34] Insiripong S, Tulayalak P, Amatachaya C. Prevalences of thalassemia/ hemoglobinopathies and G-6-PD deficiency in Malaria patients. *J Med Assoc Thai* 1996; 76(10): 554-558.

Chapter 6

ANTIMALARIAL RESISTANCE AND TREATMENT OF MALARIA IN CLINICAL PRACTICE IN THAILAND

ABSTRACT

The problem of drug resistance is the main problem affecting the success of malarial treatment worldwide. Southeast Asian countries including Thailand face up with the problem of antimalarial resistance at present. The details ranging from the molecular to social aspects of malarial resistance will be reviewed and presented. Also, the treatment of malaria in clinical practice in Thailand covering standard as well as alternative therapy for malaria to cope with the problem of high antimalarial resistance will be summarized in this article.

INTRODUCTION TO MALARIA TREATMENT

The concept of treatment is similar to other infections: getting rid of the pathogen or control of the infection and supportive or symptomatic treatment. In malaria, many antimalarial drugs (Table 1) are available for a long time. The selection of antimalarial drugs depends on the species and the reported resistance pattern in each setting [1]. Randomized controlled trials have not revealed any significant benefit of the artemisinin derivatives over quinine in quinine sensitive areas [2]. Also, if quinine is administered in the recommended way, the side effects are no greater than artemisinins [2]. Drug resistant is a very important problem in using of antimalrial drug, Historically, first case of chloroquine resistance was along the Thai-Combodian border in the late 1950s then Southeast Asia has played an important role as a focus for the development of drug resistance in *Plasmodium falciparum* [2]. In addition, the onset of chloroquine resistance marked the beginning of a new chapter in the history of malaria in Southeast Asia and by 1973 chloroquine finally had to be replaced by the combination of sulphadoxine and pyrimethamine (SP) as first line drug for the treatment of uncomplicated malaria in Thailand and more than 10 African countries have also switched their first line drug to other newly developed drug [3]. Farooq and Mahajan said that many molecular markers for antimalarial resistance had been identified, including pfmdr-1 and pfcrt polymorphisms associated with chloroquine resistance and dhfr and dhps polymorphisms associated with SP resistance [3]. They noted that polymorphisms in pfmdr-1 might also be associated with resistance to chloroquine, mefloquine and artemisinin [3]. An important precaution of using antimalarial drug is drug - induced hemolysis in the patients with glucose-6-phosphate dehydrogenase (G-6-PD) deficiency, which is endemic in the same area as malaria. It should be noted that G6PD status is recommended before primaquine or tafenoquine is prescribed in the endemic area [4]. However, the G6PD deficiency, on the other hand, is a protective factor for malaria [4]. Wajcman and Galacteros noted that red blood cells with low G6PD activity offer a hostile environment to parasite growth and thus an advantage to G6PD deficiency carriers [4].

Table 1 Summary on recommended dosage and side effects of common antimalarial drugs

Drug	Group	Dosage
Quinine sulphate	Quinoline derivative	10 mg salt/kg 8 hourly for seven days (plus doxycycline 100 mg daily for 7 days)
Quinine Dihydrochloride	Quinoline derivative	20 mg salt/kg base given intravenously in 5% normal saline as a once-only 4 hour infusion followed, 4 hours later, 10 mg salt/kg base 4-hour infusions, 8 hourly.
Chloroquine	Quinoline derivative	4 tablets (600mg base) or 10 mg/kg first dose then 2 tablets (300mg base) or 5 mg/kg 6-8 hours later for 3 days (continue with primaquine 3.5mg/kg given as a divided daily dose over 14 days)
Artesunate	Artemesin derivative	120mg intravenously stat. 60 mg at 4, 24 and 48 hours, 50-60 mg on days 3-5
Artemeter	Artemesin derivative	2 mg/kg intramuscularly stat then 1.6mg twice daily for 3-7 days

In additional to specific treatment, the supportive and symptomatic treatment is also important in taking care of malarial patients. Since several associated systemic complications like hypoglycemia, hypovolemia, hyperpyrexia, renal failure, bleeding disorders, anemia, lactic acidosis and pulmonary oedema may contribute in the pathogenesis of coma, and are responsible for high mortality, the meticulous supportive care along with intravenous administration of antimalarial drugs are corner-stone of the treatment [5]. Pamba and Maitland noted that reduction in case fatality could only come through the wider appreciation of the need for and application of supportive therapies to treat the life-threatening complications of malaria [6]. In severe malarial infection, fluid management is very important. Pamba and Maitland said that hypovolaemia had emerged as a common feature of children presenting with severe malaria complicated by acidosis [6]. They noted that early recognition and prompt treatment might lead to improvements in outcome [6]. As soon as the patient is clinically stable and able to swallow, oral treatment should be given and the intravascular volume should be maintained at the lowest level sufficient for adequate systemic perfusion to prevent development of acute respiratory distress syndrome [7]. In addition, renal replacement therapy should be initiated early [7]. Therapeutic red cell-exchange (TREX) has been used with much interest over the years to correct severe anemia [7 - 8]. Singhal said that the role of exchange blood transfusion in the management of severe malaria was still controversial and it might be considered in the presence of high parasites counts, more than10%, with multiorgan dysfunction if adequate quantities of safe blood were available [2].

Drug Resistance in Malaria

The problem of drug resistance is the main problem affecting the success of malarial treatment worldwide. The details ranging from the molecular to social aspects of malarial resistance will be reviewed and presented.

A. Molecular Aspect of Malarial Drug Resistance

The malarial drug resistance is believe to be due to the natural selection process of the parasite. A modest increase in the range of antimalarial drugs approved for clinical use has been complemented by a more impressive expansion in the analysis and understanding of the molecular mechanisms underlying resistance to these agents [9]. It is widely assumed in genetics that most mutations disrupt metabolism to some extent, and are consequently likely to be disadvantageous for the organisms that inherit them [10]. This may apply to mutations encoding drug resistance in malaria, where the mutation may be disadvantageous in the absence of the drug, imposing a genetic "cost" of resistance [10]. Many resistance mutations have rather few independent origins [11]. Although several genetic mechanisms have been described, the major source of drug resistance appears to be point mutations in protein target genes [12]. Clinically significant resistance to these agents requires the accumulation of multiple mutations, which genetic studies of parasite populations suggest arise focally and sweep through the population [12]. De novo mutation appears to be less important than migration for introducing resistance alleles into parasite populations [11]. Attempts to manage drug resistance will be of limited effectiveness unless this is taken into account [11].

Antifolate antimalarial drugs interfere with folate metabolism, a pathway essential to malaria parasite survival [13]. This class of drugs includes effective causal prophylactic and therapeutic agents, some of which act synergistically when used in combination [13]. Unfortunately, the antifolates have proven susceptible to resistance in the malaria parasite. Resistance is caused by point mutations in dihydrofolate reductase and dihydropteroate synthase, the two key enzymes in the folate biosynthetic pathway that are targeted by the antifolates [13]. Mechanisms of resistance other than reduced binding of inhibitors to mutant enzymes may be possible and need to be further explored [14]. New synergistic combinations of drugs targeting dihydrofolate reductase and dihydropteroate synthase may be employed, with new provisions against development of resistance [14].

At present, there are many advances on identification of molecular markers that can be employed in predicting in vitro and in vivo resistance in southeast Asia. Recent achievements include the successful expression of the *Plasmodium falciparum* chloroquine resistance transporter gene, pfcrt, in yeast, the identification of polymorphisms on the gamma-glutamylcysteine synthetase gene, ggcs, as potential determinants of chloroquine and mefloquine resistance, and the usefulness of a combined Plasmodium falciparum dihydrofolate reductase gene, pfdhfr, 59ARG and Plasmodium falciparum dihydropteroate synthase gene, pfdhps, 540GLU marker in reliably representing resistance to antifolates [15]. Moreover, treatment with sulfadoxine-pyrimethamine in the presence of pfdhfr 108ASP alone delayed parasite clearance and increased [15 - 16].

B. Biochemical Aspect of Malarial Drug Resistance

Ever increasing drug resistance by *P. falciparum*, the most virulent of human malaria parasites, is creating new challenges in malaria chemotherapy [17]. Applied to Plasmodium, proteomics combines high-resolution protein or peptide separation with mass spectrometry and computer software to rapidly identify large numbers of proteins expressed from various stages of parasite development [17]. Proteomic methods can be applied to study sub-cellular localization, cell function, organelle composition, changes in protein expression patterns in response to drug exposure, drug-protein binding and validation of data from genomic annotation and transcript expression studies [17]. Recent high-throughput proteomic approaches have provided a wealth of protein expression data on *P. falciparum*, while smaller-scale studies examining specific drug-related hypotheses are also appearing [17]. For new drug development, Aspects of the parasite glycolytic pathway, nucleotide metabolism, proteases, redox metabolism and organelle function have been used to highlight possible targets and molecules that could inhibit their function [18].

C. Clinical Aspect of Malarial Drug Resistance

Malarial drug resistance becomes an important problem in treatment of malaria at present. The factors which identify patients at risk of treatment failure were characterized in 1590 children and adults with uncomplicated falciparum malaria treated with 15 or 25 mg/kg of mefloquine on the borders of Thailand [19]. Six independent predictors of failure were identified using multiple logistic regression. Age < or = 2 years, 3-15 years, vomiting < 30 min after a single dose of 25 mg/kg (despite re-administration of the dose) and diarrhoea after treatment were the strongest predictors of failure by day 7 [19]. Parasitaemias > 10 000/mm^3, and fever with a history of recent vomiting (OR 1.6) were risk factors for recrudescence of the infection between days 10 and 28 [19]. At present, the distribution of antimalrial resistant malaria from Southeast Asia to other regions of the world can be seen. Recently, et al studied Chloroquine resistant malaria in neonates [20]. According to this work [20], intrauterine growth retardation, hemolytic jaundice and history of fever in the mother in the last trimester of pregnancy in the congenital while fever, history of blood transfusion in the neonates in acquired malaria but pallor in both congenital and acquired malaria groups, were important clinical features [20]. However, pattern of chloroquine resistance and mortality in congenital and acquired malaria groups was not statistically different [20].

As previously described, the genetic adaptation to the antimalarial drug of parasite as the natural selection process is considered to be the root cause of drug resistant malaria. Indeed, self-medication with anti-malarial drugs is widespread, and chloroquine resistance is increasing. In 2005, Evans et al reported the extensive prior chloroquine use in the patients presenting with severe malaria, and a high prevalence of parasites with the chloroquine - resistance genotype [21]. They noted that chloroquine resistance in *P. falciparum* might contribute to the development of severe but otherwise uncomplicated anemia [21].

D. Social Aspect of Malarial Drug Resistance

Despite more than 100 years since Laveran described plasmodium species and Ross confirmed that they were transmitted by female anopheline mosquitoes, malaria remains a leading cause of morbidity and mortality worldwide [22]. Although the areas where transmission takes place have reduced, and they are by now confined to the inter tropical areas, the number of people living at risk has grown to about 3 billions, and is expected to go on increasin [22]. With the malpractice in using of insecticide as well as self-prescribed antimalarial drug use, the problem of malarial drug resistance is widely distributed. Of interest, most of the endemic sites with the problem are the far distance rural area with limited resources. This can affect the success in treatment and control of drug resistant malaria.

Problems of Malarial Drug Resistance in Thailand

Southeast Asian countries including Thailand face up with the problem of antimalarial resistance at present. Here, the treatment of malaria in clinical practice in Thailand covering standard as well as alternative therapy for malaria to cope with the problem of high antimalarial resistance will be summarized.

A. Clinical Practice for Treatment of Drug Resistant Malaria in Thailand

For standard treatment of drug resistant malaria in Thailand, the summarized recommendation is presented in Table 2. This recommendation is proved to be useful for managing the problem of high prevalence of drug resistant malaria in Thailand.

Table 2 Simplified guideline for selection of antimalarial drugs

Species	Recommendation
Vivax	Chloroquine (Increased Dose) And Primaquine
Falciparum	Quinine dihydrochloride (intravenous)
Ovale	Similar To Vivax
Malariae	Chloroquine

* dosage of each drug is adjusted according to the recommendation of each setting

In additional to standard treatment, there are a number of researches on alternative medicine for treatment of malaria. Several herbs are tested for the possibility in development of new antimalarial drug. However, there is no herb that can be successful processed to be the real antimalarial drug for clinical use.

B. Epidemiology of Antimalarial Resistance in Thailand

Drug-resistant falciparum continues to be an increasing problem in Thailand. The high endemicity of drug resistant malaria can be seen in Western and Northern Region of Thailand , next to Myanmar. *P. falciparum* has rapidly developed resistance to new synthetic antimalarial drugs and rapidly spread by uncontrolled population movement in country and inter country. National Malaria Control Program has enforced the different strategies to overcome malaria such as disease management, drug control, in vivo and in vitro monitoring, vector control and collaboration with neighboring country. However, all of these efforts will be successful, only with community participation [23].

References

[1] Farooq U, Mahajan RC. Drug resistance in malaria. *J Vector Borne Dis*. 2004 Sep-Dec;41(3-4):45-53.

[2] Singhal T. Management of severe malaria. *Indian J Pediatr*. 2004 Jan;71(1):81-8.

[3] Indonesian Society of Medicine. Consensus of Malaria Management 2003 (part 2). *Acta Med Indones*. 2004 Jul-Sep;36(3):187-93

[4] Wajcman H, Galacteros F. Glucose 6-phosphate dehydrogenase deficiency: a protection against malaria and a risk for hemolytic accidents. *C R Biol*. 2004 Aug;327(8):711-20

[5] Garg RK. Cerebral malaria. *J Assoc Physicians India*. 2000 Oct;48(10):1004-13.

[6] Pamba A, Maitland K. Fluid management of severe falciparum malaria in African children. *Trop Doct*. 2004 Apr;34(2):67-70.

[7] Trampuz A, Jereb M, Muzlovic I, Prabhu RM. Clinical review: Severe malaria. *Crit Care*. 2003 Aug;7(4):315-23.

[8] Valbonesi M, Bruni R. Clinical application of therapeutic erythrocytapheresis (TEA). *Transfus Sci*. 2000 Jun;22(3):183-94.

[9] Hyde JE. Drug-resistant malaria. *Trends Parasitol*. 2005 Nov;21(11):494-8.

[10] Hastings IM, Donnelly MJ. The impact of antimalarial drug resistance mutations on parasite fitness, and its implications for the evolution of resistance. *Drug Resist Updat*. 2005 Feb-Apr;8(1-2):43-50

[11] Anderson TJ, Roper C. The origins and spread of antimalarial drug resistance: lessons for policy makers. *Acta Trop*. 2005 Jun;94(3):269-80.

[12] Arav-Boger R, Shapiro TA. Molecular mechanisms of resistance in antimalarial chemotherapy: the unmet challenge. *Annu Rev Pharmacol Toxicol*. 2005;45:565-85.

[13] Gregson A, Plowe CV. Mechanisms of resistance of malaria parasites to antifolates. *Pharmacol Rev*. 2005 Mar;57(1):117-45.

[14] Yuthavong Y. Basis for antifolate action and resistance in malaria. *Microbes Infect.* 2002 Feb;4(2):175-82.

[15] Wernsdorfer WH, Noedl H. Molecular markers for drug resistance in malaria: use in treatment, diagnosis and epidemiology. *Curr Opin Infect Dis*. 2003 Dec;16(6):553-8.

[16] Uhlemann AC, Krishna S. Antimalarial multi-drug resistance in Asia: mechanisms and assessment. *Curr Top Microbiol Immunol*. 2005;295:39-53.

[17] Cooper RA, Carucci DJ. Proteomic approaches to studying drug targets and resistance in Plasmodium. *Curr Drug Targets Infect Disord*. 2004 Mar;4(1):41-51.

[18] Pattanaik P, Raman J, Balaram H. Perspectives in drug design against malaria. *Curr Top Med Chem*. 2002 May;2(5):483-505.

[19] Kuile FO, Luxemburger C, Nosten F, Thwai KL, Chongsuphajaisiddhi T, White NJ. Predictors of mefloquine treatment failure: a prospective study of 1590 patients with uncomplicated falciparum malaria. *Trans R Soc Trop Med Hyg*. 1995 Nov-Dec;89(6):660-4.

[20] Khichi QK, Channar MS, Wairraich MI, Butt A. Chloroquine resistant malaria in neonates. *J Coll Physicians Surg Pak*. 2005 Jan;15(1):34-6.

[21] Evans JA, May J, Tominski D, Eggelte T, Marks F, Abruquah HH, Meyer CG, Timmann C, Agbenyega T, Horstmann RD. Pre-treatment with chloroquine and parasite chloroquine resistance in Ghanaian children with severe malaria. *QJM*. 2005 Nov;98(11):789-96.

[22] Guinovart C, Navia MM, Tanner M, Alonso PL. Malaria: burden of disease. *Curr Mol Med*. 2006 Mar;6(2):137-40.

[23] Vichaikatthaka S. The spread or drug-resistant malaria in Thailand and strategy to control. *Thai J Health Res* 1997; 13(1): 39-49.

Chapter 7

INDOCHINA AND MAE KHONG MALARIA

ABSTRACT

Indochina is a famous area of Southeast Asia. It covers Vietnam, Laos, Cambodia and northeastern part of Thailand. This area passes a long history of war.

Also, it is considered as an area with high public health and social problems. In this article, the situation and items relating to malaria in Indochina and Mae Khong will be discussed.

INTRODUCTION TO INDOCHINA

Indochinese Peninsula or Indochina is a region in Southeast Asia. It lies roughly east of India, south of China, culturally influenced by both. It covers Vietnam with the Chinese influence and Cambodia, Laos and Thailand with the Indian influence. This area passes a long history of war. A very famous Vietnam warfare occurred in this area. In addition, a long national crisis within Cambodia also occurred in Indochina. A huge of refugees were migrated from this area away from problems to the nearby countries especially Thailand and transfer to the third Western countries [1]. Also, it is considered as an area with high public health and social problems [2]. Malaria is one of the most important tropical infections in this area. Of interest, the drug resistance of malaria is also firstly mentioned from this area. In this article, the situation and items relating to malaria in Indochina and Mae Khong will be discussed.

IMPORTANT PROBLEMS OF MALARIA IN THE INDOCHINA

A. Malaria and Warfare

Although the peace happen in Indochina at present it is valuable to record and present the situation in that period. U.S. military reported for many cases of malaria in soldiers during Vietnam warfare [3]. Indeed, malaria is usually an important health problem in the foreign soldiers fighting in the endemic area. The infectious disease challenges of war include pathogens endemic to the geographic area of operations as well as wound infections with common environmental microorganisms [4]. Malaria has had a major influence on military campaigns for thousands of years. In According to a recent report, the infections in war include gastroenteritis; respiratory infection; war wound infection with antibiotic-resistant, gram-negative bacteria; Q fever; brucellosis; and parasitic infections, such as malaria and leishmaniasis [5]. Beadle and Hoffman said that the spread of drug-resistant strains of *P. falciparum*, the emergence of chloroquine-resistant *P. vivax*, and the increasing resistance of Anopheles mosquitoes to insecticides, malaria continues to be an enormous threat to U.S. Navy and Marine Corps personnel deployed to the tropics and subtropics [6]. The national military should have a powerful arsenal of educational courses and materials, personal protective measures, and malaria surveillance and control techniques in place to fight malaria in addition to enemy [7].

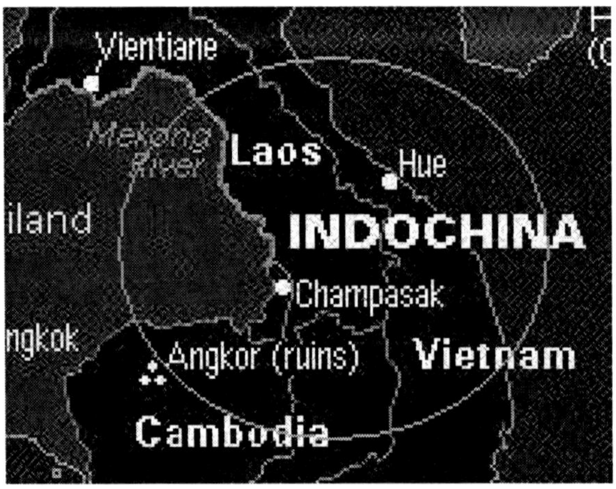

Figure 1. Indochina area.

B. Malaria and other Endemic Mae Khong Infections

In addition to malaria, there are also other tropical infectious diseases with specifically high endemic occurrence in Indochina. Here, the correlation between malaria and some important local endemic infections will be discussed. The first infection that should be mentioned is the opisthorchiasis. Opisthorchiasis or liver fluke infection is an intestinal parasite infection. The highest incidence is reported in the Indochina, especially in the area called the Emerald triangle – the area between Southern Laos, Eastern Cambodia and the Eastern most part of Thailand. Of interest, there is no report on the possible correlation between malaria and liver fluke infection. There is only an observation that elevation of soluble interleukin 2 receptor (IL-2R) in the serum can be seen in both malaria and opisthorhciasis [8]. Another local endemic infection in this area is the schistosomiasis. *Schistosoma mekongi* is the blood fluke with the specific habit in Indochina [9]. The recent discovery that individuals living in endemic areas have antibodies in their sera that are crossreactive for both helminth and malaria parasites raises important questions both of the interpretation of existing immunoepidemiological data and of the basic biology of the host and the parasites [10]. Finally, meliodosis is the bacterial infection with the highest prevalence in Indochina should also be discussed. Melioidosis is caused by the gram-negative bacillus, *Burkholderia pseudomallei* [11]. The overall mortality from this infection remains extremely high despite recent advancement in its treatment [11]. The disease, may it be acute or chronic, will be symptomatically confused with malaria, typhoid fever, leptospirosis, septicemia caused by other gram-negative bacteria, tuberculosis and mycotic infections [12]. Although there is no exact clinical report on the correlation between malaria and melioidosis it is necessary to differentiate diagnosis between these two diseases [13].

C. Malaria and Hemoglobin E

Hemoglobin E (Hb E) is the hemoglobin variant found in Indochina. It is the third common hemoglobinopathy in the world. The highest prevalence is reported in the Emerald Triangle [14]. The limited evidence for the Hb E and beta-thalassaemia mutations indicates that most have had a single origin and have subsequently reached polymorphic frequencies by selection pressure from malaria [15]. More details can be found in the chapter on natural selection and malaria.

Epidemiology of Malaria in Indochina

1. Northeastern Thailand

The northeastern part of Thailand is the previous well-known area for malaria. A region called "fire hill" in the northern part of Thailand was once the area with very high prevalence of malaria. However, the present situation of malaria is greatly reduced due to the rapid decreasing in this area. For this area, correlations between beta-globin and G-6PD genetic distances, as well as those between both sets of distances and the malarial distances, are statistically significant [16]. There is an interesting study on the frequencies of the hemoglobin E gene (HBB*E) and the beta-thalassemia gene(s) (HBB*T) in healthy adult from areas at the Thai-Kampuchean border in Northeastern Thailand [17]. According to this work, the frequencies of HBB*T were generally low, but the difference between the HBB*E frequencies in the "hills" (0.3295) and "plains" (0.2455) subgroups was highly significant and this could be interpreted as environmental effect due to selection by malaria [17]. A "hemoglobin E belt" with HBB*E frequencies between 0.3 and 0.35 extends along the Dangraek mountain chain at the border between Thailand and Kampuchea [17]. The consistently low frequencies of beta-thalassemia observed in most studied populations are explained as a result of the replacement of this genetic variant by hemoglobin E, under long-term malarial selection [16].

As previously mentioned, the drug resistance is a very important for malaria management in this area. However, Watt et al noted that oral quinine-tetracycline continued to reliably clear parasites and fever from falciparum malaria patients infected in this area of Thailand [18]. Periodic re-evaluations are warranted, however, since the decrease in vitro susceptibility to quinine may be followed by an in vivo decay in the treatment response [18]. Further details on antimalarial resistance can be found in the specific chapter in this book.

2. Central and Southern Laos

Since Loas still well preserve for the forest and wild life, malaria is still prevalence in many area of Laos. Similar to Thailand, the high prevalence of hemoglobinopathy in this area and the possible relation to malaria is also discussed. The HBB*E frequencies in the So and Alak/Ngeh tribes in Southern Laos are the highest observed in Southeast Asia in representative population samples [19]. The existence of antimalarial drug resistance in the south of Laos is confirmed and still be the important problem of malarial management in this area [20].

Of interest, there is an interesting report on the vector epidemiology of malaria in Khammouan province, Central Laos. According to the survey in, *Anopheles nivipes* accounted for more than 65% of all mosquitoes collected and was the most common species collected from human baits [21]. The results of this study show that endemic areas of malaria in Lao PDR are not necessarily related to forest [21]. Furthermore, *An. nivipes* is suspected to be the most important vector in this area [21].

3. Vietnam

Erhart et al said that although malaria has sharply decreased in Vietnam over the past 10 years, the current Health Information System (HIS) greatly underestimates the malaria burden [22]. In Vietnam, a large proportion of all malaria cases and deaths occurs in the central mountainous and forested part of the country [23]. A recent knowledge-attitude-practice survey revealed that high levels of correct knowledge about malaria's transmission and symptoms, and self-reports of adequate bed net usage and appropriate health-seeking behavior could be observed among Vietnameses [24]. Focusing on the Mae Khong delta, the reported incidence rate of clinical malaria was 2.6/100 person-years [25]. Passive case detection of clinical cases and serological follow-up of newborns carried out in a larger population confirmed the low and decreasing trend of malaria transmission [25]. However, forest malaria, despite intensive control activities, is still a major problem which raises several questions about its dynamics [23]. Luckily, a combination of insecticide-treated bednets and early diagnosis and treatment, provided free of charge, complemented by annual diagnosis and treatment during malaria surveys and community involvement with health education successfully brought malaria under control [26]. This approach could be applied to other regions in the south of Viet Nam and provides a sound basis for further studies in other areas with different epidemiological patterns of malaria [26]. In addition, involvement of the private sector and the establishment of sentinel sites might improve the quality of data and the relevance of HIS in malaria control [22].

4. Cambodia

There are around half a million cases of malaria with 5-10,000 deaths per year in Cambodia [27]. Incidence rates vary in different parts of the country [27]. Indeed, malaria has a very long history in Cambodia. In 1431, Angkor Thom, the capital of the Khmer kingdom surrendered to the Thai conquerors [28]. Soon afterwards, the young king left the city in search of a new capital [28]. As a result of the population decrease large surfaces of rice fields were abandoned and reinvaded by the jungle, the typical biotope of *An. Dirus* [28]. Severe epidemics of *P. falciparum* then occurred in the non-immune population with very high mortality decreasing again the number of workers and, thus, creating a vicious circle resulting in the progressive but complete desertion of Angkor [28].Malaria control is hampered by multiple drug resistance of *P. falciparum*, inaccessibility to the major vector, poor security in most malarious areas, and lack of resources [27]. The intercountry border areas of Thailand – Cambodia have highmalaria receptivity and vulnerability that present numerous problems in the control of malaria transmission [29]. It is thus evident that all border districts should pay more attention to control of malaria transmission and the activities of the malaria surveillance system [29]. Husum et al reported an interesting work on post injury malaria in Cambodia. Husum et al said that the rate of postinjury malaria is high despite difficulties in diagnosing postoperative malaria in endemic areas [30]. The results legitimate controlled trials of immediate postinjury chemoprophylaxis to severely injured in endemic areas and the authors also recommended staged surgical operations with brief primary interventions in victims with severe injuries [30].

5. Yunan, China

The details of the malaria situation in the Yunan region of China are available in the chapter of malaria in the Golden Triangle.

Mae Khong Malaria

The project on "Mae Khong malaria" started on 1993. The objective is to create a regional perspective in what is a global epicenter of drug resistant falciparum malaria, so to enhance the information flow required to improve malaria control on a regional basis in the context of economic and social change [31]. Geographical Information Systems technology has been applied to the regional mapping of total reported malaria cases, malaria incidence, confirmed cases, parasite species distribution [31]. Until preset, it reaches the second report. Despite the difficulties, the monograph gives confidence that the now well established collaboration is becoming a major factor in improving malaria control on a regional basis and hopefully redressing to a substantial degree the key problem of spread of drug resistance regionally and eventually globally [32].

REFERENCES

[1] Aduan RP, McCutcheon M, Eitz M, Sanger P. Refugees from Indochina. *Ann Intern Med.* 1980;92(2 Pt 1):266.

[2] Blanc F. Health report of the Indochina campaign (1945-1954). *Bull Soc Pathol Exot Filiales*. 1977;70:341-64.

[3] Porter WD. Imported malaria and conflict: 50 years of experience in the U.S. Military. *Mil Med.* 2006;171:925-8.

[4] Aronson NE, Sanders JW, Moran KA. In harm's way: infections in deployed American military forces. *Clin Infect Dis*. 2006;43:1045-51.

[5] Zapor MJ, Moran KA. Infectious diseases during wartime. *Curr Opin Infect Dis.* 2005;18:395-9.

[6] Beadle C, Hoffman SL. History of malaria in the United States Naval Forces at war: World War I through the Vietnam conflict. Clin Infect Dis. 1993;16:320-9.

[7] Robert LL. Malaria prevention and control in the United States military. *Med Trop* (Mars). 2001;61:67-76.

[8] Josimovic-Alasevic O, Feldmeier H, Zwingenberger K, Harms G, Hahn H, Shrisuphanunt M, Diamantstein T. Interleukin 2 receptor in patients with localized and systemic parasitic diseases. *Clin Exp Immunol.* 1988;72:249-54.

[9] Attwood SW. Schistosomiasis in the Mekong region: epidemiology and phylogeography. *Adv Parasitol.* 2001;50:87-152.

[10] Helmby H. Schistosomiasis and malaria: another piece of the crossreactivity puzzle. *Trends Parasitol.* 2007; [Epub ahead of print]

[11] How SH, Liam CK. Melioidosis: a potentially life threatening infection. *Med J Malaysia*. 2006;61:386-94.

[12] Kanai K, Dejsirilert S. Pseudomonas pseudomallei and melioidosis, with special reference to the status in Thailand. *Jpn J Med Sci Biol.* 1988;41:123-57.

[13] White NJ, Dance DA. Clinical and laboratory studies of malaria and melioidosis. *Trans R Soc Trop Med Hyg*. 1988;82:15-20.

[14] Trincao C. Hemoglobin E. *An Inst Med Trop* (Lisb). 1966;23:517-8.

[15] Wainscoat JS. The origin of mutant beta-globin genes in human populations. *Acta Haematol.* 1987;78:154-8.

[16] Poolsuwan S. Testing the "malaria hypothesis" for the case of Thailand: a genetic appraisal. *Hum Biol.* 2003;75:585-605.

[17] Sanguansermsri T, Flatz SD, Flatz G. The hemoglobin E belt at the Thailand-Kampuchea border: ethnic and environmental determinants of hemoglobin E and beta-thalassemia gene frequencies. *Gene Geogr*. 1987;1:155-61.

[18] Sanguansermsri T, Flatz SD, Flatz G. Quinine with tetracycline for the treatment of drug-resistant falciparum malaria in Thailand. *Am J Trop Med Hyg*. 1992;47:108-11.

[19] Flatz G, Sanguansermsri T, Sengchanh S, Horst D, Horst J. The 'hot-spot' of Hb E [beta26(B8)Glu-->Lys] in Southeast Asia: beta-globin anomalies in the Lao Theung population of southern Laos. *Hemoglobin*. 2004;28:197-204.

[20] Berens N, Schwoebel B, Jordan S, Vanisaveth V, Phetsouvanh R, Christophel EM, Phompida S, Jelinek T. Plasmodium falciparum: correlation of in vivo resistance to

chloroquine and antifolates with genetic polymorphisms in isolates from the south of Lao PDR. *Trop Med Int Health.* 2003;8:775-82.

[21] Kobayashi J, Somboon P, Keomanila H, Inthavongsa S, Nambanya S, Inthakone S, Sato Y, Miyagi I. Malaria prevalence and a brief entomological survey in a village surrounded by rice fields in Khammouan province, Lao PDR. *Trop Med Int Health.* 2000;5:17-21.

[22] Erhart A, Thang ND, Xa NX, Thieu NQ, Hung LX, Hung NQ, Nam NV, Toi LV, Tung NM, Bien TH, Tuy TQ, Cong LD, Thuan LK, Coosemans M, D'Alessandro U. Accuracy of the health information system on malaria surveillance in Vietnam. *Trans R Soc Trop Med Hyg.* 2007;101:216-25.

[23] Erhart A, Ngo DT, Phan VK, Ta TT, Van Overmeir C, Speybroeck N, Obsomer V, Le XH, Le KT, Coosemans M, D'alessandro U. Epidemiology of forest malaria in central Vietnam: a large scale cross-sectional survey. *Malar J.* 2005;4:58.

[24] Anh NQ, Hung le X, Thuy HN, Tuy TQ, Caruana SR, Biggs BA, Morrow M. KAP surveys and malaria control in Vietnam: findings and cautions about community research. *Southeast Asian J Trop Med Public Health.* 2005;36:572-7.

[25] Erhart A, Thang ND, Bien TH, Tung NM, Hung NQ, Hung LX, Tuy TQ, Speybroeck N, Cong LD, Coosemans M, D'Alessandro U. Malaria epidemiology in a rural area of the Mekong Delta: a prospective community-based study. *Trop Med Int Health.* 2004;9:1081-90.

[26] Hung le Q, Vries PJ, Giao PT, Nam NV, Binh TQ, Chong MT, Quoc NT, Thanh TN, Hung LN, Kager PA. Control of malaria: a successful experience from Viet Nam. *Bull World Health Organ.* 2002;80:660-6.

[27] Konchom S, Singhasivanon P, Kaewkungwal J, Chupraphawan S, Thimasarn K, Kidson C, Rojanawatsirivet C, Yimsamran S, Looareesuwan S. Trend of malaria incidence in highly endemic provinces along the Thai borders, 1991-2001. *Southeast Asian J Trop Med Public Health.* 2003;34:486-94.

[28] Denis MB, Meek SR. Malaria in Cambodia. *Southeast Asian J Trop Med Public Health.* 1992;23 Suppl 4:23-8.

[29] Denis MB, Meek SR. Malaria in Cambodia. *Southeast Asian J Trop Med Public Health.* 1992;23 Suppl 4:23-8.

[30] Husum H, Heger T, Sundet M. Postinjury malaria: a study of trauma victims in cambodia. *J Trauma.* 2002;52:259-66.

[31] Singhasivanon P. Mekong malaria. Malaria, multi-drug resistance and economic development in the greater Mekong subregion of Southeast Asia. *Southeast Asian J Trop Med Public Health.* 1999;30 Suppl 4:i-iv, 1-101.

[32] Socheat D, Denis MB, Fandeur T, Zhang Z, Yang H, Xu J, Zhou X, Phompida S, Phetsouvanh R, Lwin S, Lin K, Win T, Than SW, Htut Y, Prajakwong S, Rojanawatsirivet C, Tipmontree R, Vijaykadga S, Konchom S, Cong le D, Thien NT, Thuan le K, Ringwald P, Schapira A, Christophel E, Palmer K, Arbani PR, Prasittisuk C, Rastogi R, Monti F, Urbani C, Tsuyuoka R, Hoyer S, Otega L, Thimasarn K, Songcharoen S, Meert JP, Gay F, Crissman L, Cho-Min-Naing, Chansuda W, Darasri D, Indaratna K, Singhasivanon P, Chuprapawan S, Looareesuwan S, Supavej S, Kidson C, Baimai V, Yimsamran S, Buchachart K. Mekong malaria. II. Update of malaria, multi-drug resistance and economic development in the Mekong region of Southeast Asia. *Southeast Asian J Trop Med Public Health.* 2003;34 Suppl 4:1-102.

Chapter 8

MALARIA IN MALAYAN PENINSULA

ABSTRACT

Malayan Peninsula is an area of Southeast Asia. It covers Malaysia, Singapore and southern part of Thailand. This area has a wide range of social status. In this article, the situation and items relating to malaria in Malayan Peninsula will be discussed.

INTRODUCTION TO MALAYAN PENINSULA

Malayan Peninsula is a region in Southeast Asia. It covers Western Malaysia, Singapore and southern part of Thailand. This area has a wide range of social status.

Of interest, the wealth can be easily available in Singapore while the poor can be easily seen in Southern Thailand. Due to the nature of pure tropical climate, the tropical infection is important public health problem in Malayan Peninsula. In this article, the situation and items relating to malaria in Malayan Peninsula will be discussed.

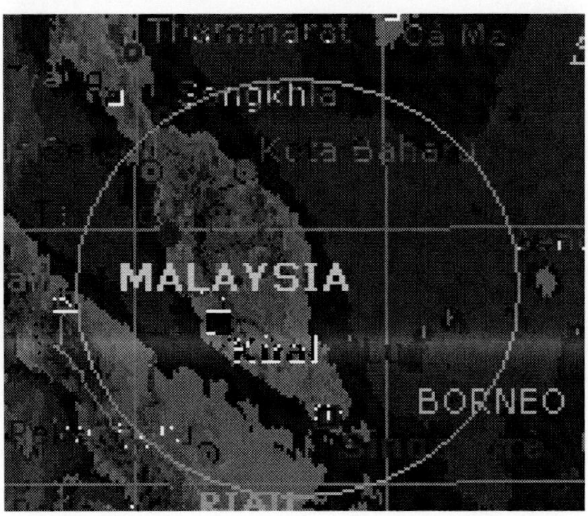

Figure 1. Malaysian Peninsula

Important Problems of Malaria in the Malayan Peninsula

A.. Malaria and Terrorism

At present, one of important local problems in the southern part of Thailand and northern part of Western Malaysia is the terrorism. The relation of malaria to the terrorism is somehow mentioned. The September 11, 2001 terrorist attacks in the United States sent shock waves throughout the world [3]. The World Bank said the events of 9/11 were likely to have mid- to long-term negative effects in some countries, and donor assistance to underdeveloped countries to fight infectious diseases including malaria could be affected [1]. Malaria is mentioned as a possible agent for bioterrorism [2 – 4]. Schroeder et al proposed that microwave-assisted processing could be useful due to its speed and robust performance wherever a rapid microscopy diagnosis is required including bioterrorism was suspected [4].

B. Malaria and Filariasis

In addition to malaria, there are also other tropical infectious diseases with specifically high endemic occurrence in Malayan Peninsula. Filariasis is another important blood infection in this area. The *Brugia malayi* is the nematode that is the main cause of filariasis in this area. Basically, the filariasis is another important mosquito borne infection in this area. A high prevalence of both malaria and filariasis in a same community can be seen [5 – 6]. An epidemiological survey of filariasis and malaria in Banggi Island and Upper Kinabatangan, Sabah, revealed microfilarial rates of 7.2% and 8.6% respectively and malaria prevalence of 9.7% and 16.9% respectively [7]. In addition, both diseases can also share the same vectors. Chang et al proposed that *Anopheles leucosphyrus*, *An. barbirostris* and *An. donaldi* were the vectors for malaria and bancroftian filariasis in forest areas of Malaysia [8]. Furthermore, the coinfection between malaria and filariasis is also reported. Graham proposed that filariasis could upset a delicate immunological balance in malaria infection and exacerbated malaria-induced immunopathology [9].

C. Malaria and Rubber tree

The Malayan Peninsula is the area where the rubber trees are commonly grown for local rubber manufacturing. It can be said that this area has the most number of rubber trees in the world. During the past three decades almost half of the existing natural tropical forests in Thailand were destroyed and replaced by cash crops, rubber, coffee, fruit orchards (durian, rambutan, mangosteen) and other commercial plantations [10]. However, malaria is still persist in Malayan Peninsula.

Singhasivanon et al proposed that new commercial plantations could provide a significant site of malaria transmission in addition to the forest and foothills areas in Southeast Asia where efficient vectors such as *An. dirus* and *An. minimus* were prevalent and had adapted to such changed ecosystems [10]. This ecological change may reintroduce malaria to a wide area [11].

EPIDEMIOLOGY OF MALARIA IN INDOCHINA

Southern Thailand

Malaria can still be detected in the southern part of Thailand although the incidence is not as high as in the north. The bionomics of Anopheles maculatus complex and its role in malaria transmission were conducted in Pakchong and Sadao districts, Nakhon Ratchasima and Songkhla provinces, respectively, from January 1984 to July 1985 [12]. According to this study, the prevalence of mosquitoes was influenced by monthly rainfall, relative humidity and air-temperature. All species of female *An. maculatus* complex studied preferred to feed on animal rather than on human, and tended to bit human more outdoors than indoors, and thus exhibiting a zoophilic and exophagic behavior [12].

Malaysia

Malaysia is a developing country with a range of parasitic infections. Indeed, soil-transmitted helminths and malaria parasites continue to have a significant impact on public health in Malaysia [13]. Until today, malaria is still one of the most important diseases in Malaysia. This is because Malaysia is located within the equatorial zone with high temperatures and humidities, usually important for the transmission of malaria [14]. The number of malaria cases were estimated to be around 300,000 before the launching of the Malaria Eradication Program (MEP) [14]. Since then and up to 1980, there was a reduction in the number of reported malaria cases from 160,385 in 1966 to 9,110 cases for Peninsular Malaysia [15]. Imported cases of malaria from nearby and distance countries to Malaysia are also reported [16]. Nine mosquito species have been reported as vectors for malaria in Malaysia: *An. maculatus*, *An balabacensis*, *An. dirus*, *An. Letifer*, *An. campestris*, *An. sundaicus*, *An. donaldi*, *An. leucophyrus* and *An. Flavirostris* [14].

Singapore

Although Singapore is a country in Malayan Peninsula area with the monsoon type climate there is no forest in this small island country. In addition, a very good sanitation in this island is accepted. Malaria is primarily an imported disease in Singapore [17]. Local outbreaks are uncommon. However, there are some sporadic localized outbreaks. Oh et al performed a study to evaluate the clinical presentation and outcome of imported malaria in Singparore [18]. According to this study, *P. vivax* is the most common cause of imported malaria, with the majority acquired from the Indian subcontinent [18]. Only a few patients presented with severe malaria [18]. In 2003, Chiam et al described a localized outbreak of three patients with Falciparum malaria, which believed to be locally acquired [17]. In this outbreak, there was one fatality due to severe disease and late presentation [17].

4. Indonesia

The northern part of Indonesia is next to Malayan Peninsula. Therefore, a similar geographical pathology to Malayan Peninsula can be expected. From epidemiological point of view, Indonesia is an extremely interesting area owing its insular structure and ecological, anthropological, cultural and economical diversity [19]. As everywhere, vector-borne diseases are the result of complex and variable epidemiological systems, subject both to biogeographical rules and human activity [19]. The major island group of Java-Bali and the remainder of the archipelago called the Outer Islands still face the malarial problem [20]. In the First National Five Year Development Plan it was changed to the Malaria Control Program with the aim to reduce the morbidity and mortality rates through surveillance and spraying interventions using the primary health care approach [21]. In 1984 in Central Java there were malaria areas with an average annual parasite incidence (API) between 1 and 7.5 promille covering about six million population, nearly one third of the population of Central Java [21]. Despite the booming of travel industry in Bali, malaria is still persistent there [22]. There are many case reports of acquired malaria from Bali [23 – 25]. The malarial prophylaxis for non immune travelers to this area is recommended [26].

REFERENCES

[1] Ssemakula JK. The impact of 9/11 on HIV/AIDS care in Africa and the Global Fund to Fight AIDS, Tuberculosis, and Malaria. *J Assoc Nurses AIDS Care*. 2002;13:45-56.

[2] Global distribution of infectious diseases requiring intensive care. Crit Care Clin. 2006;22:469-88, ix.

[3] Kirsch L. Beyond bioterrorism. *PDA J Pharm Sci Technol*. 2002;56:113-4.

[4] Schroeder JA, Gelderblom HR, Hauroeder B, Schmetz C, Milios J, Hofstaedter F, Isturiz RE, Torres J, Besso J. Microwave-assisted tissue processing for same-day EM-diagnosis of potential bioterrorism and clinical samples. *Micron*. 2006;37:577-90.

[5] Yap LF, Ramachandran CP, Balasingam E. A parasitological study of Pulau Pinang and Pulau Perhentian Kechil, off Trengganu, West Malaysia. I. Malaria and filariasis. *Med J Malaya*. 1968;23:118-22.

[6] Neo CB, Cheah YK, Chin PW, Tan TV, Wong NC, Yap LM, Kan SP. Prevalence and distribution of intestinal and blood parasites among Ibans in the Nanga Atoi in the Second Division in Sarawak. *Med J Malaysia*. 1987;42:294-8.

[7] Hii J, Kan S, Pereira M, Parmar SS, Campos RL, Chan MK. Bancroftian filariasis and malaria in island and hinterland populations in Sabah, Malaysia. *Trop Geogr Med*. 1985;37:93-101.

[8] Chang MS, Doraisingam P, Hardin S, Nagum N. Malaria and filariasis transmission in a village/forest setting in Baram District, Sarawak, Malaysia. *J Trop Med Hyg*. 1995;98:192-8.

[9] Graham AL, Lamb TJ, Read AF, Allen JE.Malaria-filaria coinfection in mice makes malarial disease more severe unless filarial infection achieves patency. *J Infect Dis*. 2005;191:410-21.

[10] Singhasivanon P, Thimasarn K, Yimsamran S, Linthicum K, Nualchawee K, Dawreang D, Kongrod S, Premmanisakul N, Maneeboonyang W, Salazar N. Malaria in tree crop plantations in south-eastern and western provinces of Thailand. *Southeast Asian J Trop Med Public Health.* 1999;30:399-404.

[11] Rosenberg R, Andre RG, Somchit L. Highly efficient dry season transmission of malaria in Thailand. *Trans R Soc Trop Med Hyg.* 1990;84:22-8.

[12] Upatham ES, Prasittisuk C, Ratanatham S, Green CA, Rojanasunan W, Setakana P, Theerasilp N, Tremongkol A, Viyanant V, Pantuwatana S, et al. Bionomics of Anopheles maculatus complex and their role in malaria transmission in Thailand. *Southeast Asian J Trop Med Public Health.* 1988;19:259-69.

[13] Singh B, Cox-Singh J. Parasites that cause problems in Malaysia: soil-transmitted helminths and malaria parasites. *Trends Parasitol.* 2001;17:597-600.

[14] Rahman WA, Che'Rus A, Ahmad AH. Malaria and Anopheles mosquitos in Malaysia. *Southeast Asian J Trop Med Public Health.* 1997;28:599-605.

[15] Lim ES. Current status of malaria in Malaysia. Southeast Asian J Trop Med Public *Health.* 1992;23 Suppl 4:43-9.

[16] Sidhu PS, Ng SC. A retrospective study on malaria cases admitted to the University Hospital, Kuala Lumpur, 1984-1988. *Med J Malaysia.* 1991;46:177-82.

[17] Chiam PT, Oh HM, Ooi EE. Localised outbreak of Falciparum malaria in Singapore. *Singapore Med J.* 2003;44:357-8.

[18] Oh HM, Kong PM, Snodgrass I. Imported malaria in a Singapore hospital: clinical presentation and outcome. *Int J Infect Dis.* 1999;3:136-9.

[19] Rodhain F. The state of vector-borne diseases in Indonesia. *Bull Soc Pathol Exot.* 2000;93:348-52.

[20] Arbani PR. Malaria control program in Indonesia. *Southeast Asian J Trop Med Public Health.* 1992;23 Suppl 4:29-38.

[21] Pribadi W, Rukmono B, Santoso SS, Soeripto N, Lokollo DM, Soeharyo. Decrease of malaria morbidity with community participation in central Java. *Southeast Asian J Trop Med Public Health.* 1992;23:389-96.

[22] Stafford EE, Sudomo M, Masri S, Brown RJ. Human parasitoses in Bali, Indonesia. *Southeast Asian J Trop Med Public Health.* 1980;11:319-23.

[23] Munckhof WJ, Grayson ML, Turnidge JD. Malaria acquired in Bali. *Med J Aust.* 1995;162:223.

[24] Ward MS, Crawford GP. Malaria acquired in Bali. Med J Aust. 1995;162:557, 560.

[25] Munckhof WJ, Grayson ML, Turnidge JD. Malaria acquired in Bali. *Med J Aust.* 1995;163:111.

[26] Grayson ML, McNeil JJ. Preventive health advice for Australian travellers to Bali. *Med J Aust.* 1988;149:462-6.

Chapter 9

ROLES OF GENOMICS AND PROTEOMICS IN MALARIA TREATMENT AND PREVENTION

ABSTRACT

Malaria is an important tropical vector borne diseases. It is one of the most problematic infectious diseases in human history. Continuous effort in development of treatment and prevention of malaria has been set for a long time. Due to the present advance medical science, genetics and molecular biology of malaria is well understood and enter into the post genomics era. Based on the advance bioinformatics and nanomedicine, genomics and proteomics gave the new way for treatment and controlling malaria. The three factors in transmission of malaria: host, agent and vector, are focused in the treatment and prevention of malaria. In addition, many recent researches applying the bioinformatics technology concerning therapeutic agent as well as vaccine for malaria are reported. Concerning the host factor, there are several studies on the genetic response to malaria infection. Modification of disease responses by other concomitant disorders such as the hemoglobinopathies as well as enzymatic deficiencies are noted. Red blood cell itself is also widely studied for the cellular genetics in metabolic change according to the infection. Host response, host susceptibility and pathogen resistance can be more clarified by the in silico investigation. Concerning the agent factor, malarial parasites of different species have been studied for their genetics. Application of bioinformatics, such as the studies of genomics epidemiology, epigenomics as well as metabolomics, help better understand the variability in malarial invasive rate and drug resistance. Concerning the vector factor, the transmission pattern of vector host mosquito can be evaluated based on the genetic pattern. In addition, studies on the genomics epidemiology accompanied with environmental parameters can help planning the control of malaria. For effective treatment of malaria, the application of several bioinformatics techniques such as chemoinformatics and quantum chemical analysis help better understand pharmacological reaction of antimalarial drug. In addition, based on the genomics and proteomics information on host, agent and drug, new drug that can solve the drug resistance, the big problem in malaria treatment, is expected. For effective prevention, application of genetic modification in the vector is the new trend. Vaccination development for malaria based on the genomics and proteomics data on malaria brings new hope in malaria prevention.

INTRODUCTION TO MALARIA

Malaria is a mosquito-borne parasitic infection. It can be said that malaria is a very important tropical mosquito-borne infectious disease. Human malaria is caused by four protozoan parasites of the genus Plasmodium: *Plasmodium*, *Plasmodium falciparum*, *Plasmodium vivax*, *Plasmodium ovale* and *Plasmodium malariae* can produce the human disease in its various forms. In human, malaria is an important is a potentially deadly mosquito-borne disease characterized by cyclical bouts of fever with muscle stiffness, shaking and sweating in the tropical countries [1 – 2]. Despite continuous effort in development of treatment and prevention of malaria has been set for a long time, the rates of disease may be re-emerging in many tropical and non-tropical countries as evidence from an increased annual parasite index. According to the globalization at present, the malaria becomes an emerging infectious problem not only to the tropical but also to the non-tropical countries. Angell and Cetron said that high-risk illnesses in travelers included childhood vaccine-preventable illnesses, hepatitis A and B, tuberculosis, malaria, and typhoid fever [3]. In addition, the problem of drug resistant malaria is increase at present. Wernsdorfer and Wernsdorfer noted that drug resistance of malaria was the most formidable obstacle in the fight against the disease since it jeopardized the most elementary objective of malaria control, namely the elimination of mortality and the reduction of suffering from malaria [4].

The mosquito vector for malaria is *Anopheles* spp. Members of 5 anopheline species complexes, *Anopheles dirus*, *Anopheles minimus*, *Anopheles sandicus*, *Anopheles aconitus* and *Anopheles manculatus*, considered to be primary malaria vectors, are also common in many tropical countries. Like all other mosquitoes, the anophelines breed in water, and each species having its preferred breeding grounds, feeding patterns and resting place [5]. Their sensitivity to insecticides is also highly variable [5]. Concerning the life cycle, Plasmodium develops in the gut of the mosquito and is passed on in the saliva of an infected insect each time it takes a new blood meal [5]. The parasites are then carried by the blood in the victim's liver where they invade the cells and multiply [5]. After 9-16 days they return to the blood and penetrate the red cells, where they multiply again, progressively breaking down the red cells [5].

The bioecological parameters, which were of special importance in the epidemiology of malaria, include three factors: host, agent and vector. These factors are the main consideration in treatment and prevention of malaria. Due to the present advance medical science, genetics and molecular biology of malaria is well understood and enter into the post genomics era. Based on the advance bioinformatics and nanomedicine, genomics and proteomics gave the new way for treatment and controlling malaria. In addition, many recent researches applying the bioinformatics technology concerning therapeutic agent as well as vaccine for malaria are reported. The knowledge on the malaria is, therefore, an interesting topic for general practitioners all over the world. There are a lot of effluxes of the knowledge from application of bioinformatics in malariology. Some interest reports on those applications are presented in this article.

FROM GENOMICS TO POST GENOMICS ERA OF MALARIA

Similar to other diseases, the studies on the genomics of malaria is believed to be the clue for the success in treatment and prevention of this disease. Coppel et al said that malaria research was dominated by information flowing from the genome sequencing projects and the associated transcriptome- and proteome-mapping projects [6]. They also noted that as more species were sequenced, comparative and phylogenetic comparisons were improving the quality of gene finding, and were providing various approaches to the identification of genes important to parasite biology and the pathogenesis of disease [6].

Due to the recent blooming of molecular biology, the genome project for malaria was launched [7 - 9]. Of several species, the *Plasmodium falciparum*, the most serious and problematic species have been widely studied. The *Plasmodium falciparum* genome project was found in 1996 by an international consortium, with support from private and government agencies in both the UK and the US [8] with the main purpose that the success of the *Plasmodium* genome project would ultimately be determined by how rapidly and effectively the information it produces is utilized by the research community to advance understanding of malaria [7]. Also, it is expected that effective dissemination of genomic information should accelerate the development of new therapeutics and vaccines [7]. According to this project, PLASMODIUM: falciparum Genome Database (PlasmoDB) (http://PlasmoDB.org) was developed [7]. This database integrates sequence information, automated analyses and annotation data emerging from the *Plasmodium falciparum* genome sequencing consortium [7]. The data (genomic DNA sequence; microsatellite and physical mapping information; predicted translations, protein features and motifs, GO classifications; BLAST results; EST, STS or GSS sequences; expression data from microarray and SAGE analyses; and newly emerging proteomics data) was accommodated from numerous *Plasmodium* and/or relevant apicomplexan species, focusing on the malarial parasite *Plasmodium falciparum* (strain 3D7; with some additional data from strains B8 and FCR3) [7, 9]. Data in PlasmoDB are organized by chromosome (1-14), and can be accessed using a variety of tools for graphical and text-based browsing or downloaded in various file formats [7, 9] (Table 1).

This work of the consortium that had been formed to complete the entire sequence of the genome of a selected clone of the human malaria parasite, Plasmodium falciparum, was finished in 2002 [10]. After that huge tracts of the genome are available as fully assembled chromosomes or large contigs and the work of initial annotation is in an advanced state [10]. Waters said that post-genomic research was in one sense the process of furthering the process of annotation, creating biological atlases and preliminary attempts to make global descriptions of gene transcription and proteome analysis were underway [10]. Waters noted that comparison between significant amounts of genome data from both closely, and more distantly related organisms, could facilitate the identification of genes themselves, coordinately regulated gene expression groups, gene function and genome organization [10]. Waters also mentioned that models of malaria could fulfill the functions and in addition provide an experimental system wherein predictions could be tested and basic experimental investigations performed within numerous aspects of disease, pathology, parasite-host and parasite-vector interactions [10]. Waters concluded that these roles would be illustrated by example and used as the basis for a discussion of the utility of genome information and malaria models in realizing the desired product of Plasmodium genomics, the development of malaria therapies [10].

Table 1. Four main area releases of PlasmoDB [7, 9].

Areas	Brief description
1. GUS (Genomics Unified Schema)	The GUS section of PlasmoDB is a relational database containing draft and finished genomic sequence, ESTs, genes and gene predictions, along with a variety of automated analyses such as predicted GO function and similarities to Pfam and ProDom domains. Graphical views of genomic sequence are available in both GIF and Java applet form. The web interface also permits Boolean combinations of query results, allowing users to combine selected queries by intersection or union.
GenePlot	The *P.falciparum* GenePlot database is a stand-alone platform-independent compilation of all available finished and unfinished DNA sequence for the *Plasmodium falciparum* genome. Contig sequence data are organized by chromosome. Annotated sequences provide links to feature indices (gene names) contained on each sequence or contig, and graphical displays of the annotated features.
Data Mining/Download	This section of PlasmoDB provides an additional set of web-based tools emphasizing data mining from unfinished and unannotated sequence. Download the current and past versions of contig sequence data. All available genomic DNA sequence data from the various sequencing centers involved in the *Plasmodium falciparum* genome project is available for retrieval, on a whole genome or chromosome-specific basis. Multiple sequence formats are provided (Fasta, GenBank, EMBL). . Where available, the nucleotide sequences and predicted coding sequence for processed RNAs can also be downloaded. BLAST results provide a hot-linked graphical interface, and links to identified sequences, facilitating further examination and analysis by the user. There are also additional Text based queries.
Links	Listing of links for malaria researchers to a variety of useful resources, including the centers responsible for generating *Plasmodium falciparum* sequence data and annotation: Sanger Centre: (http://www.sanger.ac.uk/Projects/P_falciparum/); Stanford University (http://sequence-www.stanford.edu/group/malaria/index.html); Malaria Foundation (http://www.malaria.org/); NCBI Malaria Genetics and Genomics page (http://www.ncbi.nlm.nih.gov/Malaria/); Malaria Database: (http://www.wehi.edu.au/MalDB-www/who.html); Malaria Antigen Database (http://ben.vub.ac.be/malaria/mad.html) and Rodent Malaria Index: (http://www.ncbi.nlm.nih.gov/Malaria/Rodent/index.html)

BIOINFORMATICS FOR BETTER KNOWLEDGE IN PATHOPHYSIOLOGY OF MALARIA

A. Knowledge on Host Factor: Roles of Genomics and Proteomics

Concerning the host factor, there are several studies on the genetic response to malaria infection. Basically, genetic is one of important intrinsic factors and the mechanisms controlling the ability of vectors to transmit pathogen [11]. Several studies indicate a highly polygenic basis for susceptibility to the disease, with some emerging examples of interaction between variants of specific polymorphic host and pathogen genes. Modification of disease responses by other concomitant disorders such as the hemoglobinopathies as well as enzymatic deficiencies are noted. Red blood cell itself is also widely studied for the cellular genetics in metabolic change according to the infection. The effect of genetic polymorphism in human in susceptibility and resistance of disease is proposed. May and Horstmann said that certain human genetic variants occurred only in areas endemic for malaria [12]. May and Horstmann noted that these variants protected against fatal malaria complications and cause inhibition of growth or development of malaria parasites in vitro [12]. Among these are the hemoglobins (Hb) S and C, alpha-thalassaemias, glucose-6-phosphate dehydrogenase deficiency, as well as a deletion in the erythrocyte band 3 protein [12]. Clegg and Weatherall said that the thalassemia was believed to provide protection against malaria, as a natural selection process selection to sickle cell, and it is thought that, in malarial regions of the world, natural selection had been responsible for elevating and maintaining their gene frequencies [13]. They mentioned that population and molecular genetic analysis of thalassemia variants, and microepidemiological studies of the relationship between alpha-thalassemia and malaria in the southwest Pacific, had provided unequivocal evidence for protection [13]. In addition, some of this protection appeared to derive from enhanced susceptibility in very young thalassemic children to both *Plasmodium falciparum* and, especially, *Plasmodium vivax*, and this early exposure appeared to provide the basis for better protection in later life [13]. Hb S occurs in high frequency in Africa where previously exposed to falciparum malaria [14]. Heterozygosity for the mutant sickle hemoglobin confers protection from severe *Plasmodium falciparum* infection [15]. Hebbel said that that this protection derived from the instability of sickle hemoglobin, which clustered red cell membrane protein band 3 and triggered accelerated removal by phagocytic cells [15]. Evidence for similar protective effects has been obtained for HbD and HbE, glycophorins A and C as well as for a number of immunologically relevant molecules such as human leukocyte antigens, tumor-necrosis-factor a and the inducible nitric oxide synthase [12]. Chotivanich *et al* said that HbAE erythrocytes have an unidentified membrane abnormality that renders the majority of the RBC population relatively resistant to invasion by *Plasmodium falciparum* [16]. Chotivanich *et al* said that this would not protect from uncomplicated malaria infections but would prevent the development of heavy parasite burdens and was consistent with the "Haldane" hypothesis of heterozygote protection against severe malaria for hemoglobin E [16]. Wiwanitkit also noted that the predilection occurrence of this Hb Tak in the northern region of Thailand might reflect to the natural selection process to response to the local biological hazard especially malaria [17]. These protective genetic variants indicate that malaria in endemic areas has caused a substantial selection of the human genome [17].

Concerning the roles of bioinformatics application on this point, Weatherall et al said that an analysis of the human genome with respect to variable susceptibility to infection provided important new insights into the mechanisms of human diversity [18]. Host response and host susceptibility can be more clarified by the in silico investigations. Proteins on the surface of parasite-infected erythrocytes (PIESPs) have been one of the major focuses of malaria research due to their role in pathogenesis and their potential as targets for immunity and drug intervention [19]. In 2004, Florens et al used proteomics technique to study the PIESPs on malaria infected red blood cell and could identify two novel surface proteins [19]. According to this study, these two proteins were fractionated through biotin-streptavidin interaction and analyzed by shotgun proteomics and the surface location of both proteins was confirmed by confocal microscopy using specific antibodies [19]. Florens et al concluded that in contrast to other known PIESPs, such as PfEMP1 and Rifin, these novel proteins were encoded by single copy genes, highly conserved across Plasmodium ssp., making them good targets for interventions with a broad specificity to various *Plasmodium falciparum* isolates [19]. In addition to the studies on the PIESP, there are many interesting studies to search for human genes involved in clinical malaria.

Sakunthabhai recently performed a systematic genome screening linkage analysis using genetic markers dirtributed over the human genome in order to find genes involves in genetic susceptibility to clinical malaria [20]. In this study, genomic sequences and more genetic markers were identified through the Human Genome Database and bioinformatics and the genes located in the regions were identified from database, using bioinformatics [20]. Additional search for polymorphisms was also performed with special focus on those appearing as likely candidates, based on their known function [20].

B. Knowledge on Agent Factor: Roles of Genomics and Proteomics

Scientists have now amassed a great body of knowledge about the malarial parasite [21]. Hoffman mentioned that integrated analyses of genome sequence, DNA polymorphisms, and messenger RNA and protein expression profiles will lead to greater understanding of the molecular basis of host-parasite interactions and provided strategies to build upon these insights to develop interventions to mitigate human morbidity and mortality from malaria [21]. Similar to host, the genetic diversity of the malaria itself also affect the infection. There are several studies on the genetic variations of important genes among different malarial parasites. For example, Escalante et al had investigated the genetic diversity of the gene encoding the apical membrane antigen-1 (AMA-1) in natural populations of *Plasmodium falciparum* from western Kenya and compared it with parasite populations from other geographic regions [22]. According to this study, a total of 28 complete sequences from Kenya, Thailand, India, and Venezuela field isolates were obtained and Escalante et al found that the genetic polymorphism is not evenly distributed across the gene, which was in agreement with the pattern reported in earlier studies [22]. They also reported an evidence supporting limited gene flow between the parasite populations, specifically, between the Southeast Asian and Venezuelan isolates but no alleles could be linked to a specific geographic region [22]. Escalante et al had also investigated the genetic diversity of the gene encoding the transmission-blocking vaccine antigen Pfs48/45 of *Plasmodium falciparum* parasites from western Kenya and compared it with parasite populations from Thailand, India, and Venezuela [23]. They found that the Pfs48/45 gene of Kenyan parasites was more polymorphic than parasites from other geographic origins and they mentioned that positive natural selection was involved in the maintenance of the observed polymorphism [23].

The genome of plasmodium itself is also widely investigated by the database mining and functional analysis technique in order to find the new drug targets. Cowman recently performed a study to identify a number of families of genes encoding proteins that appear to play a role in the invasion of the merozoite form of *Plasmodium falciparum* into human red blood cells by the mentioned techniques [24]. According to their study, the erythrocyte binding antigen 175 and the reticulocyte binding proteins, similar to those identified in Plasmodium vivax, can be detected [24]. In addition, further functional analysis of these proteins using reverse genetic confirmed their role in invasion [24]. In 2005, Healer et al used the functional analysis approach to analyze of Plasmodium falciparum apical membrane antigen 1 utilizing interspecies domains, a leading malaria vaccine candidate whose function has not been unequivocally defined [25]. They reported that specific chimeric AMA1 proteins containing domains I to III from PfAMA1 and PcAMA1 were able to complement PfAMA1 function in erythrocyte invasion [25]. They also demonstrated that domain III did not contain dominant epitope targets of antibodies raised against Escherichia coli expressed and refolded PfAMA1 ectodomain. In additional, they generated a parasite line in which the N-terminal pro region of PfAMA1 did not undergo proteolytic cleavage and show that its removal is necessary for PfAMA1 function [25].

Application of bioinformatics, such as the studies of genomics epidemiology, gene expression, epigenomics as well as metabolomics, help better understand the variability in malarial invasive rate and drug resistance. The genomics epidemiology of resistant strain malaria is focused in the new pharmacological study [26]. As previous mentioned, there are several genetic diversities of malaria such as those described in AMA-1 and Pfs48/45 [22 – 23].

Indeed, resistance of malarial parasites to antifolates suchs as pyrimethamine and cycloguanil is known to be due to multiple mutations of dihydrofolate recutase (DHFR) [27]. Recently, et al sued proteomic technique to explore the mechanisms that may potentiate the antifolate resistance in addition to decreased drug binding of mutant enzymes [27]. According to this study, they noted that comparatives studies of protein expression profiles of four parasite strains of Plasmodium falciparum carrying wild-type (TM4/8.2) DHFR enzymes revealed several proteins spots that were differentially expressed [27]. In order to study the expression of the malaria, several algorithms have been proposed. In 2005, Simpson et al performed a comparison of match-only algorithms for the analysis of Plasmodium falciparum oligonucleotide arrays [28].

In this study, they compared the performance of three match-only algorithms on these data: the Match Only Integral Distribution (MOID) algorithm, Robust Multichip Analysis (RMA), and the Model Based Expression Index (MBEI) and validated the differential expression of several genes using quantitative reverse transcriptase-PCR [28]. They found similar performance of those algorithms [28]. In additional to gene expression analysis, epigenetics is one of the key areas of future research that can elucidate how genomes work and it combines genetics and the environment to address complex biological systems such as the plasticity of the genome. While all nucleated cells carry the same genome, they express different genes at different times. For malaria, epigenetic phenomena can also be seen. Recently, Scherf et al employed a selective panning protocol to generate isogenic Plasmodium falciparum populations with defined adhesive phenotypes for CD36, ICAM-1 and CSA, expressing single and distinct var gene variants [29]. In this study, they established the framework for examining var gene expression, its regulation and switching and it was found that var gene switching occured in situ and ubiquitous transcription of all var gene variants appeared to occur in early ring stages, however, var gene expression is tightly regulated in trophozoites and is exerted through a silencing mechanism [29]. In this study, in situ var gene switching is apparently mediated at the level of transcriptional initiation, as demonstrated by nuclear run-on analyses [29]. Scherf et al suggest that an epigenetic mechanism was involved in var gene regulation [29].

In the post-genomic era, the application of the knowledge of malarial parasite metabolism is widely discussed. Using metabolomics technique, the metabolic pathway of the parasite has been mapped based on the current knowledge of parasite biochemistry and on the pathways known to occur in eukaryotes. Some of the metabolic pathways are significantly different from the host such as hemoglobin degradation and lipid biosynthesis [30]. Krungkrai noted that understandings of metabolic functions will illuminate new chemotherapeutic targets, including known targets for antimalarial drugs in currently used [30]. Krungkrai said that the pyrimidine enzymes of the parasite might be monofunctional forms while the host had five enzymes associated into two different multifunctional proteins [30]. Generally, DHFR is a critical target associated with antifolate resistance in malaria. Efforts have therefore been devoted to determine the three dimensional structure of the plasmodium DHFR, in order to use for further docking study which can provide more knowledge on the interaction of DHFR and its inhibitor at atomic levels. There are several studies on this topic. Recently, Lemcke et al used homology building technique to construct a three-dimensional (3-D) model of DHFR from *Plasmodium falciparum* [31]. In this study, the 3-D model of the plasmodial DHFR was obtained by amino acid substitution in the human DHFR, which was chosen as template, modification of four loops (two insertions, two deletions) and subsequent energy minimization [31]. According to this study, the significance of the most important point mutation causing resistance, S108N, could be explained by the model, whereas the point mutations associated with enhanced resistance, N51I and C59R, seem to have a more indirect effect on inhibitor binding [31]. In 2002, Chitnumsab et al reported the successful crystallization of the DHFR. According to this study, a full-length pfdhfr-ts gene was clonded from the genomic DNA of *Plasmodium falciparum* and inserted into a modified pET (17b) plasmid [32. Further study on the expression, characterization and crystallization of *Plasmodium falciparum* bifunctional DHFR-thymidylate synthethase was performed [32]. Yavaniyama et al also performed additional study on the X-ray structure of the DHFR-thymidylate synthethase complex and found that a crystal of the complex belong to the $P2_12_12_1$ spacegroup with cell parameters equal to 59.98, 157.10 and 164.61 angstrom, respectively [33].

C. Knowledge on Vector Factor: Roles of Genomics and Proteomics

Presently, there are many studied about the role of the vector genetic in the diffusion of malaria. Conclusively, population genetic studies of vectors are essential for (a) the determination of their taxonomic status and consequently the definition of their vectorial role in the transmission of pathogenic agents; (b) the evaluation of the species genetic variability and the estimation of their capacities of adaptation to selection pressure; (c) an estimation of gene flow among populations in order to evaluate their degree of isolation and gene circulation, especially resistance genes [34]. The transmission pattern of vector host mosquito can be evaluated based on the genetic pattern. In addition, studies on the genomics epidemiology accompanied with environmental parameters can help planning the control of malaria. The *Anopheles gambiae* genome sequence, together with the recent development of molecular tools for genome-wide analysis, promises new insights into the biology of the malaria vector [35]. Morlais et al said that these insights should help define the best possible breakdown point for interrupting transmission in the mosquito vector [35]. Morlais et al performed a survey of the intraspecific nucleotide diversity in coding regions of three different mosquito strains showed an average of one single nucleotide polymorphism (SNP) every 125 coding base pairs [35]. According to this study, high levels of nucleotide polymorphism were observed in mosquito immune-related genes and pathogen recognition receptors harbored higher replacement substitutions and genotyping at SNP loci in natural populations of *Anopheles gambiae* from three malaria foci showed contrasting patterns [35]. They also found that the distribution of mutation Y443H in the thioester-containing protein 3 (TEP3) gene suggested this mutational event had occurred under selective constraints [35]. In 2005, Kriventseva et al presented an analysis of 215,634 EST and cDNA sequences of a major vector of human malaria *Anopheles gambiae* structured into the AnoEST, a vital resource for interpretation of expression profiles derived using recently developed *Anopheles gambiae* cDNA microarrays, database [36]. In this study, the expressed sequences were grouped into clusters using genomic sequence as template and associated with inferred functional annotation, including the following: corresponding Ensembl gene prediction, putative orthologous genes in other species, homology to known proteins, protein domains, associated Gene Ontology terms, and corresponding classification into broad GO-slim functional groups [36]. Using these cDNA microarrays, Kriventseva et al have experimentally confirmed the expression of 7,961 clusters during mosquito development and found that 3100 were not associated with currently predicted genes [36]. They also found that clusters with confirmed expression were nonbiased with respect to the current gene annotation or homology to known proteins and proposed that many as yet unconfirmed clusters were likely to be actual *Anopheles gambiae* genes [36].

New Antimalarial Drug, Vaccine and Transgenic Vector for Malaria: New Ways for Malaria Treatment and Control

New Antimalarial Drug

The concept of treatment is similar to other infections: getting rid of the pathogen or control of the infection and supportive or symptomatic treatment. In malaria, many antimalarial drugs are available for a long time. Drug resistant is a very important problem in using of antimalrial drug, Historically, first case of chloroquine resistance was along the Thai-

Combodian border in the late 1950s then Southeast Asia has played an important role as a focus for the development of drug resistance in *Plasmodium falciparum* [37]. In addition, the onset of chloroquine resistance marked the beginning of a new chapter in the history of malaria in Southeast Asia and by 1973 chloroquine finally had to be replaced by the combination of sulphadoxine and pyrimethamine (SP) as first line drug for the treatment of uncomplicated malaria in Thailand and more than 10 African countries have also switched their first line drug to other newly developed drug [37]. Farooq and Mahajan said that many molecular markers for antimalarial resistance had been identified, including pfmdr-1 and pfcrt polymorphisms associated with chloroquine resistance and dhfr and dhps polymorphisms associated with SP resistance [37]. They noted that polymorphisms in pfmdr-1 might also be associated with resistance to chloroquine, mefloquine and artemisinin [37].

To cope with the increase problem of the antimalarial resistance parasite, there is a requirement for searching for new drugs as well as new drug targets. For effective treatment of malaria, the application of several bioinformatics techniques such as chemoinformatics and quantum chemical analysis help better understand pharmacological reaction of antimalarial drug. Recently, Yuthavong et al developed novel analogs of pyrimethamine and cyclogaunil as inhibitors of antifolate resistant Plasmodium falciparum bearing multiple mutations of DHFR and tested these compounds for the binding and inhibition properties [38]. According to this study, three are several compounds with good antimalarial activities and can be the alternative for new drug development [38]. In additional to development of new drug, quantumchemical analysis can help better understand of the present available antimalarial drug. In 2002, Tonmunphean et al used the quantum chemical analysis to study the reaction mechanism of artemisinin compound and its relation to antimalarial activity. According to this study, they found that homolytic C-C clevage reaction was energetically and was more preferable that the intramolecular hydrocarbon shift process [39]. In additional, the relationships between antimalarial activity and the calculated energies were also detected [39].

Vaccine

Concerning the vaccination for malaria, there are many interesting recent reports on this topic. Tongren *et al* said that it had been repeatedly argued that the discovery and implementation of a safe and effective vaccine against malaria was a major priority in the control of the disease [40]. Concerning transgenic vector for controlling of malaria, engineering mosquitoes with a genetic trait that confers resistance to malaria or causes population suppression is a task [41]. In addition, chemoprophylaxis of malaria is recommended for the traveler entering malarial endemic area [42]. In addition, chemoprophylaxis is also highly effective in reducing mortality and morbidity from malaria in young children and pregnant women living in endemic areas [43]. Greenwood said that intermittent preventive treatment, in which full therapeutic doses of a drug are given at defined intervals, had the potential to provide some of the benefits of sustained chemoprophylaxis in pregnant women and young children without some of its drawbacks and was a promising new approach to malaria control [43]. Hatz said that exposure prophylaxis substantially reduced the risk of infection [44]. Drugs for chemoprophylaxis is indicated. Petersen said that use of malaria chemoprophylaxis was a balance between the risk of infection and death, and the risk of side effects [45]. Three levels of chemoprophylaxis are used: chloroquine in areas with sensitive *Plasmodium falciparum*, chloroquine plus proguanil in areas with low level chloroquine resistance, and atovaquone/proguanil, doxycycline or mefloquine in areas with extensive resistance against chloroquine and proguanil [45]. Hatz also noted that if malaria infection was readily diagnosed, the infection could always be successfully treated [44].

To develop a vaccine for malaria, many advances in bioinformatics have to be applied. The modeling as well as epitope structural analysis is needed. Kinetic analysis of the resistant mutant can help find active site residue. Doolan et al said thatrecent advances in the fields of genomics, proteomics and molecular immunology offer tremendous opportunities for the development of novel interventions against public health threats, malaria [46]. However, they said that effectively identify the targets of protective T cell or antibody responses from genomic data was not available and the identification of antigens that would stimulate the most effective immunity against the target pathogen is problematic, particularly if the genome was large : the 23 Mb *Plasmodium falciparum* genome encodes more than 5,300 proteins, each of which was a potential target of protective immune responses [46]. Therefore, advance search from improving the computational epitope searching tools is necessary. In additional, the possible target epitope has to be further tested for the inhibitory ctivity. Recently, Uthaipibull et al studied the merozoite surface protein (MSP-1), a prime candidate for malaria vaccine development [47]. This protein has inhibitory activity that can prevent the secondary proteolytic processing step and inhibit erythrocyte invasion, however, it also has blocking activity, which blocks both the previous described inhibition activity and red blood cell invasion [47]. The neutralizing and blocking properties of this protein and its recombinants was studied [47].

CONCLUSION

At present, there is lot of new knowledge in malariology. The application of new genomics and proteomics can help better understand the pathophysiology of the disease. In additional, several bioinformatics techniques are applied for new studies in treatment and prevention of malaria (Table 2)

Table 2. Some important applications of bioinformatics technologies in malariology

Purpose	Example of applications
Mining for new basic Knowledge	Database development Sequence analysis Structural analysis
Treatment	Functional and expression analysis Chemoinformatics Quantum chemistry
Prevention	Molecular modeling and docking Epitope analysis Molecular modeling and docking

REFERENCES

[1] Chareonviriyaphap T, Bangs MJ, Ratanatham S. Status of malaria in Thailand. *Southeast Asian J Trop Med Public Health* 2000; 31: 225-37.

[2] Phillips RS. Current status of malaria and potential for control. *Clin Microbiol* 2001; 14: 208 – 26.

[3] Angell SY, Cetron MS. Health disparities among travelers visiting friends and relatives abroad. *Ann Intern Med* 2005; 142: 67-72.

[4] Wernsdorfer G, Wernsdorfer WH. Malaria at the turn from the 2nd to the 3rd millenium. *Wien Klin Wochenschr* 2003; 115 Suppl 3: 2-9.

[5] Ladhani S, El Bashir H, Patel VS, Shingadia D. Childhood malaria in East London. *Pediatr Infect Dis J* 2003; 22: 814-9.

[6] Coppel RL, Roos DS, Bozdech Z. The genomics of malaria infection. *Trends Parasitol* 2004;20:553-7.

[7] PlasmoDB: An integrative database of the Plasmodium falciparum genome. Tools for accessing and analyzing finished and unfinished sequence data. The Plasmodium Genome Database Collaborative. *Nucleic Acids Res* 2001; 29:66-9.

[8] Fletcher C. The Plasmodium falciparum Genome Project. Parasitology Today 1998; 14: 342–344.

[9] Bahl A, Brunk B, Coppel RL, Crabtree J, Diskin SJ, Fraunholz MJ, Grant GR, Gupta D, Huestis RL, Kissinger JC, Labo P, Li L, McWeeney SK, Milgram AJ, Roos DS, Schug J, Stoeckert CJ Jr. PlasmoDB: the Plasmodium genome resource. An integrated database providing tools for accessing, analyzing and mapping expression and sequence data (both finished and unfinished). *Nucleic Acids Res* 2002;30:87-90.

[10] Waters AP. Orthology between the genomes of Plasmodium falciparum and rodent malaria parasites: possible practical applications. *Philos Trans R Soc Lond B Biol Sci* 2002;357:55-63.

[11] Paul RE, Day KP. Mating Patterns of Plasmodium falciparum. *Parasitol Today.* 1998;14:197-202.

[12] May J, Horstmann R. Influence of human genetic variants on resistance and immunity against malaria. *Bundesgesundheitsblatt Gesundheitsforschung Gesundheitsschutz* 2004; 47 :1000-8.

[13] Clegg JB, Weatherall DJ. Thalassemia and malaria: new insights into an old problem. *Proc Assoc Am Physicians* 1999; 111: 278-82.

[14] Roberts DJ, Williams TN. Haemoglobinopathies and resistance to malaria. *Redox Rep* 2003; 8: 304-10.

[15] Hebbel RP. Sickle hemoglobin instability: a mechanism for malarial protection. *Redox Rep.* 2003; 8: 238-40.

[16] Chotivanich K, Udomsangpetch R, Pattanapanyasat K, Chierakul W, Simpson J, Looareesuwan S, White N. Hemoglobin E: a balanced polymorphism protective against high parasitemias and thus severe P falciparum malaria. *Blood* 2002; 100: 1172-6.

[17] Wiwanitkit V. Haemoglobin Tak, an unstable haemoglobin from Thailand. *Haema* 2004; 7: 310-312.

[18] Weatherall D, Clegg J, Kwiatkowski D. The role of genomics in studying genetic susceptibility to infectious disease. *Genome Res* 1997;7:967-73.

[19] Florens L, Liu X, Wang Y, Yang S, Schwartz O, Peglar M, Carucci DJ, Yates JR 3rd, Wub Y. Proteomics approach reveals novel proteins on the surface of malaria-infected erythrocytes. *Mol Biochem Parasitol* 2004;135:1-11.

[20] Sakuntabhai A. Genomics approaches in searching for genes involved in clinical malaria. Presented at the International Conference on Bioinformatics 2002. Bangkok Thailand, 2002

[21] Hoffman SL, Subramanian GM, Collins FH, Venter JC. Plasmodium, human and Anopheles genomics and malaria. *Nature* 2002;415:702-9.

[22] Escalante AA, Grebert HM, Chaiyaroj SC, Magris M, Biswas S, Nahlen BL, Lal AA. Polymorphism in the gene encoding the apical membrane antigen-1 (AMA-1) of Plasmodium falciparum. X. Asembo Bay Cohort Project. *Mol Biochem Parasitol* 2001;113:279-87.

[23] Escalante AA, Grebert HM, Chaiyaroj SC, Riggione F, Biswas S, Nahlen BL, Lal AA. Polymorphism in the gene encoding the Pfs48/45 antigen of Plasmodium falciparum. XI. Asembo Bay Cohort Project. *Mol Biochem Parasitol* 2002;119:17-22.

[24] Cowman AF. Database mining and functional analysis of the Plasmodium falciparum genome sequence. Presented at the International Conference on Bioinformatics 2002. Bangkok Thailand, 2002

[25] Healer J, Triglia T, Hodder AN, Gemmill AW, Cowman AF. Functional analysis of Plasmodium falciparum apical membrane antigen 1 utilizing interspecies domains. *Infect Immun* 2005;73:2444-51.

[26] Kidson C. Malaria genomics and disease control. *Southeast Asian J Trop Med Public Health* 2002;33:669-70.

[27] Vanuchatanantkul J, Kamchonwongpaisan S, Yuthavong Y. Proteomic analysis of antifolate resistant strains of Plasmodium falciparum. Presented at the International Conference on Bioinformatics 2002. Bangkok Thailand, 2002

[28] Simpson KM, Baum J, Good RT, Winzeler EA, Cowman AF, Speed TP. A comparison of match-only algorithms for the analysis of Plasmodium falciparum oligonucleotide arrays. *Int J Parasitol* 2005;35:523-31.

[29] Scherf A, Hernandez-Rivas R, Buffet P, Bottius E, Benatar C, Pouvelle B, Gysin J, Lanzer M. Antigenic variation in malaria: in situ switching, relaxed and mutually exclusive transcription of var genes during intra-erythrocytic development in Plasmodium falciparum. *EMBO J* 1998;17:5418-26.

[30] Krungkrai J. Bioinformatics and metabolic function in malarial parasite. Presented at the International Conference on Bioinformatics 2002. Bangkok Thailand, 2002

[31] Lemcke T, Christensen IT, Jorgensen FS. Towards an understanding of drug resistance in malaria: three-dimensional structure of Plasmodium falciparum dihydrofolate reductase by homology building. *Bioorg Med Chem* 1999;7:1003-11.

[32] Chitnumsub P, Vanichtanantkul J, Yavaniyama J, Kamchonwongpaisarn S, Sirawaraporn W, Yuthavong Y. Expression, characterization and crystallization of Plasmodium falcuparum bifunctional dihydrofolate reductase-thymidylate synthase. Presented at the International Conference on Bioinformatics 2002. Bangkok Thailand, 2002

[33] Yavaniyama J, Chitnumsub P, Vanichtanantkul J, Kamchonwongpaisarn S, Taylor P, Walkinshaw MD, Sirawaraporn W, Yuthavong Y. X-ray structure determination of Plasmodium falcuparum bifunctional dihydrofolate reductase-thymidylate synthase.

Presented at the International Conference on Bioinformatics 2002. Bangkok Thailand, 2002

[34] Failloux AB, Vazeille-Falcoz M, Mousson L, Rodhain F. Genetic control of vectorial competence in Aedes mosquitoes. *Bull Soc Pathol Exot* 1999; 92: 266-73.

[35] Morlais I, Poncon N, Simard F, Cohuet A, Fontenille D. Intraspecific nucleotide variation in Anopheles gambiae: new insights into the biology of malaria vectors. *Am J Trop Med Hyg* 2004;71:795-802.

[36] Kriventseva EV, Koutsos AC, Blass C, Kafatos FC, Christophides GK, Zdobnov EM. AnoEST: Toward A. gambiae functional genomics. *Genome Res*. 2005;15:893-9.

[37] Farooq U, Mahajan RC. Drug resistance in malaria. J Vector Borne Dis 2004; 41: 45-53.

[38] Yuthavong Y, Kamchonwongpaisarn S, Vanichtanantkul J, Chitnumsub P, Jarprung D, Tarcchompoo B, Sirichaiwat C, Sirawaraporn W, Thebtaranoth Y, Lowe G. Presented at the International Conference on Bioinformatics 2002. Bangkok Thailand, 2002

[39] Tonmunphean S, Parasuk V, Kokpol S. Quantum chemical calculations on reaction mechanisms of artemisinin compounds: related with antimalarial activity. Presented at the International Conference on Bioinformatics 2002. Bangkok Thailand, 2002

[40] Tongren JE, Zavala F, Roos DS, Riley EM. Malaria vaccines: if at first you don't succeed. *Trends Parasitol* 2004; 20: 604-10 .

[41] Christophides GK. Transgenic mosquitoes and malaria transmission. *Cell Microbiol* 2005; 7: 325-: 33.

[42] Wiwanitkit V. Amazing Thailand Year 1998-1999 Tourist's health concepts. *Chula Med J* 1998; 42: 975-984.

[43] Greenwood B. The use of anti-malarial drugs to prevent malaria in the population of malaria-endemic areas. *Am J Trop Med Hyg* 2004; 70: 1-7.

[44] Hatz CF. Prophylaxis and therapy of malaria in the practice. *Internist* (Berl) 2004; 45: 677-83

[45] Petersen E. Malaria chemoprophylaxis: when should we use it and what are the options? *Expert Rev Anti Infect Ther* 2004; 2: 119-32.

[46] Doolan DL, Aguiar JC, Weiss WR, Sette A, Felgner PL, Regis DP, Quinones-Casas P, Yates JR 3rd, Blair PL, Richie TL, Hoffman SL, Carucci DJ. Utilization of genomic sequence information to develop malaria vaccines. *J Exp Biol* 2003;206:3789-802.

[47] Uthaipibull C, Fernandex-Reyes D, Feeney J, Holder A. Modelling of P. falciparum MSP1- mutants and epitope structural analysis of neutralizing and blocking antibodies. Presented at the International Conference on Bioinformatics 2002. Bangkok Thailand, 2002

Chapter 10

Biochemoinformatics Technology and Malarial Vaccine

Abstract

Biochemoinformatics is a new science that can lead several advantages in medicine. The field of vaccinology is benefit from the new technologies of bioinformatics. The complete genome sequences of malarial parasite is complete. Vaccines can now be targeted towards specific gene products that traditional vaccine research failed to discover. Advanced biochemoinformatics technologies for vaccine development can be applied for vaccine development of several diseases including to malaria.

Introduction to Biochemoinformatics

History

Several physicians of the 19th century had only a few knowledge of the transmission of some human hereditary traits [1]. Critical examination of pedigrees culminated in formulation of a "law of heredity" before the rediscovery of Mendel's classical work [1]. Genetics began when Mendel proved his laws of hereditary with varieties of peas and flowers in 1865 [2 – 4]. The first law, the law of independent segregation occurs in Mendel's paper as an assumption or hypothesis [3]. Hugo de Vries refers to this as a law discovered by Mendel. This appears to be the first use of an expression equivalent to Mendel's law [3]. The second law, the law of independent assortment, is present and also later confirmed [3]. Starting from the question of heredity, such as it was defined by Darwin in 1868, there are several development in genetics [2]. For examples of progression, the invention of the compound microscope was occurred in the 19th century. Amino acid sequencing for protein was then successful and the first complete sequencing of an enzyme, ribonuclease, was reported in 1960 [5]. After that the sequencing of the first complete genome (*Haemophilus influenzae*) published in 1995 [6].

With the feasibility to sequence an organism's genome, the giant projected call "Genome Project" was then started. In 1990, Human Genome Project (HGP) by the United States Department of Energy (DoE) and the National Institutes of Health was stared with the main goals to identify all chemical base pairs and all genes that make up the 23 chromosome pairs found in human DNA [7 - 8]. In 1988, Congress appropriated funds to the Department of Energy and the National Institutes of Health to begin planning the Human Genome Project [9]. Planners set a 15-year time frame, estimated that the price tag would be $3 billion, and laid formal goals to get the job done [9]. On October 1, 1990, the Human Genome Project officially began [9]. This work was already successful in 2001. The post genome era came after that. Since the HGP brought to light the limitations of traditional lab work although mostly automated they are expensive and time consuming, therefore, there is a need for the new technology to help solve this problem. It needs to incorporate original techniques to allow greater understanding of protein function, protein-protein interactions and protein-DNA interactions and put it all in a cellular context. An application of the computational technologies can help answer this problem.

Biochemoinformatics is the new emerged science in the postgenomic era. Bioinformatics has been split into various subjects, several "omics." Computational technologies can be fully applied in biochemoinformatics. Firstly, data mining is the first basic application of computational technologies in bioinformatics [10]. Basically, passive techniques includingvarious techniques in statistic, namely, Min, Max, SD, regression and correlation are used for graph and histogram generation. However, these techniques are out of date. New active techniques such as Artificial Intelligence (AI) are therefore generated to replace the passive ones. With the advancement in AI for active data mining, several further applications in "omic" sciences can be derived.

Bioinformatics

The word bioinformatics was first coined in 1988 by Dr. Hwa Lim and its original definition was "a collective term for data compilation, organisation, analysis and dissemination" [11]. Basically, bioinformatics uses information technology to help solve biological problems by designing novel and incisive algorithms and methods of analyses [11 – 12]. It also serves to establish innovative software and create new/maintain existing databases of information, allowing open access to the records held within those databases [11 – 12]. The first branch of bioinformatics is genomics. Genomics refers to the analysis of all of the genes and transcripts included within the genome. It starts from nucleic acid characterization [13 - 14]. The basic principles are a) all genes have certain regulatory signals positioned in or about them, b) all genes by definition contain specific code patterns, and c) many genes have already been sequenced and recognized in other organisms so we can infer function and location by homology if our new sequence is similar enough to an existing sequence. All of these principles can be used to help locate the position of genes in DNA and are often known as "searching by signal," "searching by content," and "homology inference" respectively. Many servers are established to help with gene finding analyses. Many servers combine many of the methods previously discussed consolidate the information and often combine signal and content methods with homology inference in order to ascertain exon locations [13 – 14].

At present, there several sub-branches of genomics. Complete genomic sequences are now available for many organisms/bacteria/viruses/organelles and can be used for further comparison. Analyzing and comparing genetic material from different species to study evolution, gene function, and inherited disease are the basic principle of comparative genomics [15]. It can help understand the uniqueness between different species. For comparison, gene location, gene structure (exon number, exon lengths, intron lengths and sequence similarity) as well as gene characteristics (splice sites, codon usage and conserved synteny) can be used [15]. The cross-referencing of information on genome organization between species provides an additional dimension to the Human Genome Project and can derive much information from it for the benefit of animal health and animal breeding [16]. Arrangements of genes and other DNA sequences may be determined by a variety of genetic and physical techniques, at resolutions from the gross cytological level to the level of the single base pair [16]. Information about location and function of genes is directly transferable across species and should greatly accelerate the search for genes that specify inherited diseases in domestic mammals and humans as well as genes that specify economically important traits [16].

Functional genomics is another sub-branch of genomics. Functional genomics means the development and application of genome-wide or system-wide experimental approaches to assess gene function by making use of the information and reagents provided by structural genomics. It is characterized by high-throughput or large-scale experimental methodologies combined with statistical or computational analysis of the results [17]. Many electronic and laboratory approaches are being developed to meet this challenge but the rate of evolution of these is not keeping pace with the speed of sequence generation [17 – 18]. For functional genomics, biochemical experiment and genetic method. However, this approach is out of date. In silico experiment is widely used at present. Basically, computational biology strives to extract the maximal possible information from known sequences, by classifying them according to their homologous relationships, predicting their biochemical activity, cellular function, 3-dimensional structures and evolutionary origin [17 – 18]. Computational genomics is a subfield of computational biology that deals with the analysis of entire genome sequences [19]. Transcending the boundaries of classical sequence analysis, computational genomics exploits the inherent properties of entire genomes by modeling them as systems [19]. Homology method (BLAST), Phylogenetic profile and Fusion method (Rosetta stone analysis) are the three widely used techniques in functional genomics [20]. Homology method uses searching proteins whose amino acid sequences are similar. In addition, analysis of correlated mRNA expression levels enables to establish functional linkages, by detecting changes in mRNA expression in different cell types, or different environments. Phylogenetic profile describes the pattern of presence or absence of a particular protein, across a set of organisms [21]. Features or dynamics of the evolutionary process are much more easily inferred with large numbers of taxa, and large numbers are essential for discriminating differences in evolutionary patterns between sites [21]. Accurate prediction of site-specific patterns can improve phylogenetic reconstruction by an amount equivalent to quadrupling sequence length [21]. Fusion method (Rosetta stone analysis) based on the principle that some pairs of interacting proteins have homologs in another organism, fused into a single protein chain.

Structural genomics is another sub-branch of genomics. It studies protein-protein interactions, protein recognization to its ligand, functional prediction and protein fold identification. The approach of structural genomics to study a large number of targets in parallel has been commonly applied to protein families and even whole genomes [22]. A great challenge in structural genomics era is to predict protein structure and function from sequence, including the identification of biological partners [23]. The development of a procedure to construct position-specific scoring matrices for the prediction and identification of sequences with putative significant affinity faces this challenge [23]. The local and web applications used for sequence and structure search, sequence alignment, protein modeling, molecule edition and modification, and scoring matrices construction are available [23].

In addition to genomics, proteomics is another important "omic" science in bioinformatics. Sequence alignment, looking for homology, is also important in proteomics. For proteomics, homology is defined as the divergent evolution of two proteins from a common ancestor. Solving of the structural format of protein is also important in proteomics. It is closed related to structural genomics [23].Organization of the knowledge by gene ontology technique is important for studying of a protein function. Genes in biological databases are linked to GO terms, allowing biologists to ask questions about gene function in a manner independent of species [24]. In gene ontology, biological process, molecular function and cellular component of a protein is very useful for further protein study [24]. The Gene Ontology (GO) project provides a controlled vocabulary to facilitate high-quality functional gene annotation for all species [24].

Chemoinformatics

Chemical informatics is the application of information technology to chemistry but not with a specific focus on drug discovery. Chemoinformatics encompasses the design, creation, organisation, management, retrieval, analysis, dissemination, visualization and use of chemical information [25 - 26]. Structural prediction, substructure searching and similarity searching is the basic chemoinformatics techniques. Structural, physicochemical and ADME-Tox property profiles of reference (successful) ligands, along with structural information of their target proteins, have been extremely useful for early-stage drug discovery [25 – 26]. Recently, databases of known biologically active ligands (knowledge bases) have become more focused toward different protein-target classes [25 – 26]. In addition, quantum mechanics and molecular mechanics can be applied in chemoinformatics for studying of a chemical reaction. Intramolecular energy determination is important for studying of molecular stabilization in various conformational changes. Basically, total energy is the summation of stretching energy, bending energy, torsion energy and non-bonded interactions energy. For intermolecular energy determination, reaction energy can be studied. Basically, reactions are fundamentally rearrangements of electron configurations. Mechanisms describe the specific flow of electrons, the transient intermediates, and the final products should be clarified for all biochemical reaction. Thermodynamics principle can applied for reaction mechanism study. Total requirement energy is equal to energy getting in minuses energy giving out due to bond breaking and bond formation, respectively. Given limited time and input energy, a reactions may only achieve kinetic equilibrium, settling into an energy local minimum between large activation energy barriers. Finally, the study on the complex formation can also be performed similar to bioinformatics.

VACCINE DISCOVERY BY BIOINFORMATICS TECHNIQUES

Brief History

Vaccine has been discovered and used for two centuries [27]. Although vaccines exist against almost 30 different diseases and search remains ongoing on additional new vaccines, many of the presently existing and used vaccines are distance from ideal [28]. Twenty percentage of global mortality, especially in children under the age of five is due to infectious diseases and vaccines are effective at controlling of these diseases, as shown by the success of smallpox eradication, the impressive progress towards polio eradication and the significant achievements in measles mortality [29]. A number of substantial unresolved questions cloud the current approach, and the development of vaccines against these organisms has proved very challenging [30]. New biotechnology technologies and vaccinologists are facilitating the rapid expansion of the clinical drug search, empowering clinicians with a better understanding of disease as well as novel alternatives for treating patients [31]. Many candidate vaccines have been tested in animal models [31]. The immunogenicity and the safety of some vaccine formulations have been recently tested through clinical trials, and the efficacy of these vaccine therapies in humans must be determined in the near future [31].

As for other fields of medical sciences, it is expected that vaccinology will greatly benefit from the emerging genomics technologies such as bioinformatics, proteomics and DNA microarrays [32]. The post-genomic era just starting therefore promises an exponential increase of vaccine research and new vaccines, both improved vaccines with a greater efficacy and less adverse effects to replace old ones and vaccines for prevention of diseases for which no vaccines is available [27]. The availability of complete genome sequences in combination with novel advanced technologies, have revolutionized the approach to vaccine development [33]. Current developments in computational vaccinology mainly support the analysis of antigen processing and presentation and the characterization of targets of immune response [34]. At present, vaccine technologists are using microarrays, immunoinformatics, proteomics and high-throughput immunology assays to reduce the unmanageable volume of information available in genome databases to a manageable size [35]. Immunomics is a new omics science that addresses the interface between host and pathogen proteome, bridging informatics, genomics, proteomics, immunology and clinical medicine [36]. This large-scale screening of immune processes which includes powerful immunoinformatic tools offers great promise for future translation of basic immunology research advances into successful vaccines [34].

Immunomics

The development of DNA microarray technology a decade ago led to the establishment of functional genomics as one of the most active and successful scientific disciplines today [37]. With the ongoing development of immunomic microarray technology-a spatially addressable, large-scale technology for measurement of specific immunological response-the new challenge of functional immunomics is emerging, which bears similarities to but is also significantly different from functional genomics [37]. Immunomicroarray is now the modern technique in study of many diseases [38 – 39]. Immunonic data has been successfully used to identify biological markers involved in autoimmune diseases, allergies, viral infections such as human immunodeficiency virus (HIV), influenza, diabetes, and responses to cancer vaccines [37].

Immunology research has been transformed in the post-genomics era, with high throughput molecular biology and information technologies taking an increasingly central role. The astounding diversity of immune system components together with the complexity of the regulatory pathways and network-type interactions makes immunology a combinatorial science [40 - 41]. Computational analysis has therefore become an essential element of immunology research with a main role of immunoinformatics being the management and analysis of immunological data. More advanced analyses of the immune system using computational models typically involve conversion of an immunological question to a computational problem, followed by solving of the computational problem and translation of these results into biologically meaningful answers [41]. This has led to the development of a new area of science termed "Immunomics", that encompasses genomic, high throughput and bioinformatic approaches to immunology [40].

Major immunoinformatics developments include immunological databases, sequence analysis, structure modelling, mathematical modelling of the immune system, simulation of laboratory experiments, statistical support for immunological experimentation and immunogenomics [41]. An important aspect of immunomics relating to vaccine development is the epitope prediction. T-cell-epitope mapping has emerged as one of the most powerful new drug discovery tools for a range of biomedical applications [42 - 43]. Initially, T-cell-epitope discovery was applied to the development of vaccines for - infectious diseases and cancer [42 - 43]. T-cell-epitope-mapping applications have now expanded to include reengineering of protein therapeutics (a process now called deimmunization), as well as the fields of autoimmunity, endocrinology, allergy, transplantation and diagnostics [42 - 43]. Research employing T-cell-epitope mapping falls within the realm of immunomics, a new field that addresses the interface between host and (pathogen) proteome, bridging informatics, genomics, proteomics, immunology and clinical medicine [42 - 43]. Epitope prediction is the hope of immunomics for new vaccine finding at present. The National Institute of Allergy and Infectious Diseases (NIAID), part of the National Institutes of Health (NIH), recently awarded 14 contracts to fund the Large-Scale Antibody and T Cell Epitope Discovery Program [44]. Expectation to find new vaccine based on epitope prediction via immunomics techniques is the most recent facet of vaccinology.

Bioinformatics for Malarial Vaccine Development

1. Genomics Research for Malarial Vaccine Development

Analysis of the malarial genome sequence has provided promising new leads for drug and vaccine development [45]. Identification of the targets of protective T cell or antibody responses from genomic data is the heart of analysis of genome sequence [46]. However, the identification of antigens that will stimulate the most effective immunity against the target pathogen is still problematic since the malarial genome is large. The 23 Mb *Plasmodium falciparum* genome encodes more than 5,300 proteins, each of which is a potential target of protective immune responses [46].

Comparative genomics technique is useful for determination of difference among genes encoding vaccine candidate antigens. Recently, Safitri et al studied the amino-terminal region of the serine repeat antigen (SERA) of *Plasmodium falciparum*, a major malaria-vaccine candidate [47]. In this work, they investigated the patterns of sequence diversity in exon II of SERA gene and found that sequence variation in exon II might represent one of the parasite's immune-evasion strategies [47]. Ferriera et al analyzed sequence variation in block 2 repeats and in non-repetitive block 17, as well as other polymorphisms within the merozoite surface protein-1 (MSP-1) gene, in clinical isolates of *Plasmodium falciparum* [48]. Basically, the merozoite surface protein of Plasmodium spp hass been considered as a vaccine candidate, which exhibits antigenic diversity among isolates [49]. According to this work, they indicated a role for non-homologous recombination, such as strand-slippage mispairing during mitosis and gene conversion, in creating variation in a malarial antigen under strong diversifying selection [48].

For application of structural genomics, several tools are overcoming several of the obstacles for studying protein expression in the malaria parasite, vastly accelerating the pace for antigen discovery [50]. Together, these conceptual and technological advances allow a rational approach to vaccine antigen selection, in which a finite number of antigens are selected from the entire genome by merit of the expression patterns and specific features [50]. These candidate antigens are then subjected to detailed studies according to criteria established by the understanding of pathogenesis and protective immunity, to identify the optimal antigens for inclusion in subunit vaccines [50]. In order to assess possible effects of a polymorphic vaccine, Fluck et al analyzed the genetic diversity of parasites collected in the course of a phase 2b field trial of the blood stage vaccine Combination B in Papua New Guinea [51]. The full-length 3D7 allele of the merozoite surface protein 2 (MSP2) was included in Combination B as one of three subunits [51]. Extensive genetic diversity of MSP2 was observed in both the repetitive and family-specific domains, but alleles occurring in vaccine recipients were no different from those found in placebo recipients [51]. A phylogenetic analysis showed no clustering of 3D7-type breakthrough infections from vaccine recipients [51].

2. Proteomics Research for Malarial Vaccine Development

The 23 Mb *Plasmodium falciparum* genome encodes more than 5,300 proteins, each of which is a potential target of protective immune responses [46]. However, the current generation of subunit vaccines is based only on a single or few antigens and therefore might elicit too narrow a breadth of response [46]. Proteomics and computational analysis of these databanks are being used to model and investigate the three-dimensional structure of many key malaria proteins in an attempt to facilitate vaccine design [52]. Recombinant protein expression in bacteria and yeast coupled with cGMP purification technologies and conditions have lead to the recent availability of several dozen malaria protein antigens for human-use Phase I and Phase II vaccine trials [52]. For examples of applied studies on malarial proteome, Haddad et al recently rapidly tested hundreds of DNA vaccines encoding exons from the *Plasmodium yoelii yoelii* genomic sequence [53]. Orthologs of protective

Plasmodium yoelii yoelii genes were then identified in the genomic databases of *Plasmodium falciparum* and *Plasmodium vivax* and investigated as candidate antigens for a human vaccine [53]. Identified exons were then were cloned into a DNA immunization vector with the Gateway cloning technology [53]. In this work, high-throughput cloning of exons into DNA vaccines and their screening is feasible and can rapidly identify new malaria vaccine candidate antigens [53]. In another study, Aguiar et al examined the feasibility of a high-throughput cloning approach using the Gateway system to create a large set of expression clones encoding *Plasmodium falciparum* single-exon genes [54]. In this work, master clones and their ORFs were transferred en masse to multiple expression vectors and target genes were selected using specific sets of criteria, including stage expression and secondary structure and the genes were subcloned into a DNA vaccine vector [54]. In animal model testing, the functional expression of genes to generate antibody against various stages of the parasite could be observed [54].

There are also some recent researches making used of gene ontology techniques for identification of malarial vaccine candidate proteins. Glutathione reductase (GR) is an NADPH-dependent enzyme that reduces oxidized glutathione (GSSG) to GSH. Naturally, GR is present in human and in *Plasmodium* spp. GR is also focused in malarial vaccine development. However, the function of the GR in malarial infection is not well characterized. Wiwanitkit used a new gene ontology technology to predict the molecular function and biological process [55]. Using GoFigure server, the molecular function and biological process in human and *P. falciparum* GR is predicted [55]. Comparing to the human GR, the *P. falciparum* GR has similar molecular functions as gluthathione disulfide reductase activity, oxidoreductase activity, disulfide oxidoreductase activity and metal ion binding [55]. Wiwanitkit also performed a similar study on carbonic andrydrase. A similar finding can be detected [56].

3. Immunomics Research for Malarial Vaccine Development

There are a few reports on application of immunomics for malarial vaccine development. Here, the author performed a mini-study on T-cell epitope finding as an example for immunomics study for malarial vaccine development. Malarial VAR2CSA may have value as a protective immunogen in novel vaccines [57]. The main aim of this study is to find potential T-cell epitopes of. Here, the author reports the preliminary data from the computational analysis of VAR2CSA to find potential T-cell epitopes using a new bioinformatics tool. The author performed computation analysis of available VAR2CSA of malaria type 2 sequence (accession number = ABK91145, 316 residues) to find potential T-cell epitopes using bioinformatics tool namely MHCPred (available from the URL: http://www.jenner.ac.uk/MHCPred) [58]. The MHCPred tool is a partial least squaresbased multivariate robust statistical approach to the quantitative prediction of peptide binding to major histocompatibility complexes (MHC), the key checkpoint on the antigen presentation pathway within adaptive cellular immunity [58]. MHCPred implements robust statistical models for both Class I alleles (HLA-A*0101, HLAA*0201, HLA-A*0202, HLA-A*0203, HLA-A*0206, HLA-A*0301, HLA-A*1101, HLA-A*3301, HLA-A*6801, HLA-A*6802 and HLA-B*3501) and Class II alleles (HLA-DRB*0401, HLA-DRB*0401 and HLA-DRB*0701) [58]. The results of computational analysis included peptides and their corresponding IC50 value, which implies the binding affinity. Usually, peptides with predicted binding affinities < 500 nM are good binders, whereas those with binding affinities > 5000 nM are considered non binders [59].

The alleles selected for binding affinity prediction are A0101, A0201, A0202,A0203, A0206, A0301, A1101, A3101, A6801, A6802, B3501, DRB0101, DRB0401and DRB0701. According to the analysis, peptides with the best predicted binding affinities for each studied are presented in Table 1. Among all alleles, the results from DRB0101, A0203 and A0101 show significant lower IC50 than other alleles.

Identification of epitopes capable of binding multiple HLA types will significantly rationalize the development of epitope-based vaccines [60]. In this work, the author used a new bioinformatic tool to predict potential T-cell epitopes. The technique used in this study is similar to a previous recent report [61]. The peptides with best binding affinities for each allele are determined. The determined peptides are useful for further vaccine development because it can reduce the time and minimize the total number of required tests to find the possible proper epitopes, the target for vaccine development. The design of multi-epitope vaccines can also based on these identified epitopes. Conclusively, the author used a computational analysis to determine the potential T-cell epitopes of VAR2CSA. According to this work, 40 IQKETELLY48 corresponding to DRB0101 allele is the peptide with the best binding affinity. However, some limitations of this study should be mentioned. The results from this study are only predicted results. Further confirmation is required. Further in vitro synthesis of the determined peptide and in vivo experimental study to test the efficacy are the future steps for vaccine development.

REFERENCES

[1] Lenay C. Hugo De Vries: from the theory of intracellular pangenesis to the rediscovery of Mendel. *C R Acad Sci III*. 2000;323:1053-60.

[2] Czihak G, Rassem T. Dawn of human genetics. *NTM*. 1994;2:175-82.

[3] Monaghan F, Corcos A. On the origins of the Mendelian laws. *J Hered*. 1984;75:67-9.

[4] Svob T. Mendel and Mendalism and his place in medicine. (100th anniversary of the mendelian law). *Med Arh*. 1965;19:29-40.

[5] Hirs CH, Moore S, Stein WH. The sequence of the amino acid residues in performic acid-oxidized ribonuclease. *J Biol Chem*. 1960;235:633-47.

[6] Fleischmann RD, Adams MD, White O, Clayton RA, Kirkness EF, Kerlavage AR, Bult CJ, Tomb JF, Dougherty BA, Merrick JM, et al. Whole-genome random sequencing and assembly of Haemophilus influenzae Rd. *Science*. 1995;269:496-512.

[7] Watson JD. The human genome project: past, present, and future. Science. 1990;248:44-9.

[8] Cantor CR. Orchestrating the Human Genome Project. *Science*. 1990;248:49-51.

[9] Panchal J, Brandt EN Jr. The Human Genome Research Project: implications for the healthcare industry. *J Okla State Med Assoc*. 2001;94:155-9.

[10] Bork LS. Data mining: sophisticated forms of managed care modeling through artificial intelligence. *J Health Care Finance*. 1997;23:20-36.

[11] Lim HA, Venkatesh TV. Bioinformatics in the pre- and post-genomic eras. *Trends Biotechnol.* 2000;18:133-5.
[12] Venkatesh TV, Bowen B, Lim HA. Bioinformatics, pharma and farmers. *Trends Biotechnol.* 1999;17:85-88.
[13] Ashburner M, Goodman N. Informatics--genome and genetic databases. *Curr Opin Genet Dev.* 1997;7:750-6.
[14] McKusick VA. Genomics: structural and functional studies of genomes.*Genomics.* 1997;45:244-9.
[15] O'Brien SJ, Wienberg J, Lyons LA. Comparative genomics: lessons from cats. *Trends Genet.* 1997;13:393-9.
[16] Graves JA. Background and Overview of Comparative Genomics. *ILAR J.* 1998;39:48-65.
[17] Hieter P, Boguski M. Functional genomics: it's all how you read it. *Science.* 1997;278:601-2.
[18] Rastan S, Beeley LJ. Functional genomics: going forwards from the databases. *Curr Opin Genet Dev.* 1997;7:777-83.
[19] Tsoka S, Ouzounis CA. Recent developments and future directions in computational genomics. *FEBS Lett.* 2000;480:42-8.
[20] Haubold B, Wiehe T. Comparative genomics: methods and applications. *Naturwissenschaften.* 2004;91:405-21.
[21] Pollock DD. Genomic biodiversity, phylogenetics and coevolution in proteins. *Appl Bioinformatics.* 2002;1:81-92.
[22] Lundstrom K. Structural genomics for membrane proteins. *Cell Mol Life Sci.* 2006;63:2597-607.
[23] Fernandez-Ballester G, Serrano L. Prediction of protein-protein interaction based on structure. *Methods Mol Biol.* 2006;340:207-34.
[24] Lomax J. Get ready to GO! A biologist's guide to the Gene Ontology. Brief Bioinform. 2005;6:298-304.
[25] Parker CN, Schreyer SK. Application of chemoinformatics to high-throughput screening: practical considerations. *Methods Mol Biol.* 2004;275:85-110.
[26] Ghose AK, Herbertz T, Salvino JM, Mallamo JP. Knowledge-based chemoinformatic approaches to drug discovery. *Drug Discov Today.* 2006;11:1107-14.
[27] Makela PH. Vaccines, coming of age after 200 years. *FEMS Microbiol Rev.* 2000; 24: 9-20.
[28] Combinations, the key to global immunization. *CVI Forum.* 1993; (5):2-6.
[29] Kieny MP, Girard MP. Human vaccine research and development: an overview. *Vaccine.* 2005: 23: 5705-7.
[30] Alsahli M, Farrell RJ, Michetti P. Vaccines: an ongoing promise? *Dig Dis.* 2001; 19: 148-57.
[31] Avidor Y, Mabjeesh NJ, Matzkin H. Biotechnology and drug discovery: from bench to bedside. *South Med J.* 2003; 96: 1174-86.
[32] Grandi G. Rational antibacterial vaccine design through genomic technologies. *Int J Parasitol* 2003; 33: 615-20.
[33] Capecchi B, Serruto, D., Adu-Bobie, J., Rappuoli, R., Pizza, M. The genome revolution in vaccine research. *Curr Issues Mol Biol.* 2004; 6: 17-27.

[34] Brusic V, August JT, Petrovsky N. Information technologies for vaccine research. *Expert Rev Vaccines*. 2005; 4: 407-17.

[35] De Groot AS, Rappuoli R. Genome-derived vaccines. *Expert Rev Vaccines*. 2004; 3: 59-76.

[36] De Groot AS. Immunomics: discovering new targets for vaccines and therapeutics. *Drug Discov Today*. 2006; 11: 203-9.

[37] Braga-Neto UM, Marques ET Jr. From functional genomics to functional immunomics: new challenges, old problems, big rewards. *PLoS Comput Biol*. 2006;2:e81.

[38] Mayne M, Cheadle C, Soldan SS, Cermelli C, Yamano Y, Akhyani N, Nagel JE, Taub DD, Becker KG, Jacobson S. Gene expression profile of herpesvirus-infected T cells obtained using immunomicroarrays: induction of proinflammatory mechanisms. *J Virol*. 2001;75:11641-50.

[39] Belleville E, Dufva M, Aamand J, Bruun L, Christensen CB. Quantitative assessment of factors affecting the sensitivity of a competitive immunomicroarray for pesticide detection. *Biotechniques*. 2003;35:1044-51.

[40] Brusic V, Petrovsky N. Immunoinformatics--the new kid in town. *Novartis Found Symp*. 2003;254:3-13

[41] Petrovsky N. Immunome research. *Immunome Res*. 2005;1:1.

[42] Brusic V, August JT, Petrovsky N. Information technologies for vaccine research. *Expert Rev Vaccines*. 2005;4:407-17.

[43] De Groot AS.Immunomics: discovering new targets for vaccines and therapeutics. *Drug Discov Today*. 2006;11:203-9.

[44] Sette A, Fleri W, Peters B, Sathiamurthy M, Bui HH, Wilson S. A roadmap for the immunomics of category A-C pathogens. *Immunity*. 2005;22:155-61.

[45] Gardner MJ. The genome of the malaria parasite. *Curr Opin Genet Dev*. 1999; 9: 704-8.

[46] Doolan DL, Aguiar JC, Weiss WR, Sette A, Felgner PL, Regis DP, Quinones-Casas P, Yates JR 3rd, Blair PL, Richie TL, Hoffman SL, Carucci DJ. Utilization of genomic sequence information to develop malaria vaccines. *J Exp Biol*. 2003; 206: 3789-802.

[47] Safitri I, Jalloh A, Tantular IS, Pusarawati S, Win TT, Liu Q, Ferreira MU, Dachlan YP, Horii T, Kawamoto F. Sequence diversity in the amino-terminal region of the malaria-vaccine candidate serine repeat antigen in natural Plasmodium falciparum populations. *Parasitol Int*. 2003; 52: 117-31.

[48] Ferreira MU, Ribeiro WL, Tonon AP, Kawamoto F, Rich SM. Sequence diversity and evolution of the malaria vaccine candidate merozoite surface protein-1 (MSP-1) of Plasmodium falciparum. *Gene*. 2003; 304: 65-75.

[49] Zakeri S, Dinparast Djadid N, Zeinal, S. Sequence heterogeneity of the merozoite surface protein-1 gene (MSP-1) of Plasmodium vivax wild isolates in southeastern Iran. *Acta Trop*. 2003; 88: 91-7.

[50] Duffy PE, Krzych U, Francis S, Fried M. Malaria vaccines: using models of immunity and functional genomics tools to accelerate the development of vaccines against Plasmodium falciparum. *Vaccine*. 2005;23:2235-42.

[51] Mahajan B, Noiva R, Yadava A, Zheng H, Majam V, Mohan KV, Moch JK, Haynes JD, Nakhasi H, Kumar S. Effect of the malaria vaccine Combination B on merozoite surface antigen 2 diversity. *Infect Genet Evol*. 2007;7: 44-51.

[52] Chiang PK, Bujnicki JM, Su X, Lanar DE. Malaria: therapy, genes and vaccines. *Curr Mol Med*. 2006; 6: 309-26.

[53] Haddad D, Bilcikova E, Witney AA, Carlton JM, White CE, Blair PL, Chattopadhyay R, Russell J, Abot E, Charoenvit Y, Aguiar JC, Carucci DJ, Weiss WR. Novel antigen identification method for discovery of protective malaria antigens by rapid testing of DNA vaccines encoding exons from the parasite genome. *Infect Immun*. 2004; 72: 1594-602.

[54] Aguiar JC, LaBaer J, Blair PL, Shamailova VY, Koundinya M, Russell JA, Huang F, Mar W, Anthony RM, Witney A, Caruana SR, Brizuela L, Sacci JB Jr, Hoffman SL, Carucci DJ. High-throughput generation of P. falciparum functional molecules by recombinational cloning. *Genome Res*. 2004; 14: 2076-82.

[55] Wiwanitkit V. Plasmodium and host glutathione reductase: molecular function and biological process. *African J Biotech*. 2006; 5: 2009-2013.

[56] Wiwanitkit V. Plasmodium and host carbonic anhydrase: molecular function and biological process. *Gene Ther Mol Biol Vol*. 2006; 10: 251-254.

[57] Dahlback M, Rask TS, Andersen PH, Nielsen MA, Ndam NT, Resende M, Turner L, Deloron P, Hviid L, Lund O, Pedersen AG, Theander TG, Salanti A. Epitope mapping and topographic analysis of VAR2CSA DBL3X involved in P. falciparum placental sequestration. *PLoS Pathog*. 2006;2:e124.

[58] Guan P, Doytchinova IA, Zygouri C, Flower DR. MHCPred: bringing aquantitative dimension to the online prediction of MHC binding. Appl Bioinformatics. 2003 2:63 - 6.

[59] Guan P, Hattotuwagama CK, Doytchinova IA, Flower DR. MHCPred 2.0: an updated quantitative T-cell epitope prediction server. *Appl Bioinformatics*. 2006;5:55-61.

[60] Doytchinova I, Flower D. The HLA-A2-supermotif: a QSAR definition. *Org Biomol Chem*. 2003;1:2648-54.

[61] Wiwanitkit V. Predicted epitopes of H5N1 bird flu by bioinformatics method: a clue for further vaccine development. *Chinese Med J* 2006; 119: 1760.

Chapter 11

TRAVEL, MIGRATION AND MALARIA

ABSTRACT

Malaria is still an important infectious disease in Southeast Asia. The study of the incidence of malaria can provide useful data for disease prevention and control. At present, trade and travel can impact on vector-borne diseases, including malaria Transmission of malaria from endemic area to non endemic area can be expected and this can affect the pattern of malaria epidemiology.

INTRODUCTION

Malaria is an important potentially fatal mosquito-borne disease characterizedby cyclical bouts of fever with muscle stiffness, shaking and sweatingin tropical countries including Southeast Asian countries [1]. In Thailand, organized malaria control activities have reduced malaria morbidity from 286/1000 population in 1947 to 1.5/1000 population by 1996 [2]. Despite encouraging trends in dramatically reducing malaria, the rates of disease may be re-emerging in the country as evidenced from an increase annual parasite index from 1.78/1000 in 1997 to 2.21/1000 in 19981 [2]. It can be shown that the pattern of malarial incidence is dynamic and the study of the incidence of malaria can provide useful data for disease prevention and control.Global change includes climate change and climate variability, land use, waterstorage and irrigation, human population growth and urbanization, trade and travel,and chemical pollution can impact on vector-borne diseases, including malaria [3].Transmission of malaria from endemic area to non endemic area can be expected andthis can affect the pattern of malaria epidemiology.

TRAVEL MEDICINE FOR IMPORTANT MOSQUITO BORNE INFECTIONS

Travel is an important factor causing the emerging of mosquito borne infection in a new setting [4]. Good examples are the case of dengue infection and yellow fever. In the past, North America is considered as a dengue-free region. However, dengue infection became an important imported emerging infection in recent few years. Within the last decade witnessed unprecedented global dengue epidemic activity in the American hemisphere. DeHart said that vectors for yellow fever, malaria, and dengue had been identified on aircraft and should be Considered as an important health issue of air travel [5]. Pinheiro said that the emergence of epidemic dengue hemorrhagic occurred in 1981 almost 30 years in the Americas after its appearance in Asia, and its incidence was showing a marked upward trend [6]. Pinheiro noted that a main cause of the emergence of DHF in the Americas was the failure of the hemispheric campaign to eradicate *Aedes aegypti*. Similar to North America, dengue infection has been imported into Europe for few years. Haas *et al* noted that some emerging infectious diseases including dengue infection had recently become endemic in Germany [7]. They also noted that outbreaks of dengue fever in endemic areas were reflected in increased infections in travelers returning from these areas [7]. Badiaga *et al* recently performed an interesting retrospective study on imported dengue infection in France [8]. They found that dengue infection was increasingly observed in febrile travelers returning from tropical areas,2 especially those returning from the Caribbean islands and Southeast Asia, but it was rarely diagnosed in travelers returning from Africa [8]. In a retrospective study of 44 cases of imported dengue infection diagnosed in France, Badiaga *et al* found that the epidemiologic, clinical and diagnostic characteristics of these cases were similar to those reported in other previous published studies [8]. Gascon *et al* performed another study in 57 Spanish travelers with imported dengue infection [9]. In this report, all patients had travelled to endemic areas (Central America 28 cases, Indian subcontinent 15, Southeast Asia 10, South America 2, West Africa one, and Pacific one) [9]. The following were the most important clinical characteristics: fever and asthenia (100%), headache (98%), myalgia (84%), arthralgia (72%), morbilliform rash (61%) and retroocular pain (65%) [9]. Gascon *et al* noted that dengue should be included in differential diagnosis of fever in patients coming back to travels to tropical areas [9].For yellow fever, North America is not considered as an endemic area of yellow fever. Dutch slave traders brought yellow fever to the Americas from Africa during the mid-seventeenth century [10]. For the next two and a half centuries, the disease terrorized seaports throughout the Americas [10]. Throughout the 19th century, yellow fever was the scourge of southern coastal cities [11]. However, Tomori noted that recent increases in the density and distribution of the urban mosquito vector, *Aedes aegypti*, as well as the rise in air travel increased the risk of introduction and spread of yellow fever to North America [12]. Yellow fever became an important imported emerging infection in USA in recent few years. At present, many countries require a valid international certificate of vaccination from travelers, including those in transit, arriving from infected areas or from countries with infected areas [13]. Some countries require a certificate from all entering travelers, even those arriving from countries where there is no risk of yellow fever [13]. Van Laethem said that yellow fever vaccine was the only mandatory vaccine for certain African or south American countries [14]. In many Asian countries, vaccination is strongly advised for tourist outside urban areas of endemic countries even if these countries have not officially reported the disease and do not require evidence of vaccination on entry [4,14].

Travel And Malaria

Similar to dengue infection and yellow fever, malaria is an important topic in travel medicine. Malaria becomes very important in any type of traveling including to Hajj [15]. Long-term travelers, defined here as those traveling for periods of 6 months or longer, face particular challenges regarding malaria prevention [16]. Increasing numbers of people are travelling to tropical destinations where they are at risk of malaria [17]. A prevention traditionally relies on chemoprophylaxis during and after exposure [18]. Long-term travelers have a higher risk of malaria than short-term travelers. Long-term travelers underuse personal protective measures and adhere poorly to continuous chemoprophylaxis regimens [16]. The risk of side effects from chemoprophylaxis needs to be balanced against the risk of infection [18]. A number of strategies are used during long-term stays: discontinuation of chemoprophylaxis after the initial period, sequential regimens with different medications for chemoprophylaxis, stand-by emergency self-treatment, and seasonal chemoprophylaxis targeting high-incidence periods or locations [16]. Three levels of chemoprophylaxis are used: chloroquine in areas with sensitive P. falciparum, chloroquine plus proguanil in areas with low level chloroquine resistance, and atovaquone/proguanil (Malarone, GlaxoSmithKline), doxycycline or mefloquine (Lariam, Roche) in areas with extensive resistance against chloroquine and proguanil [19]. Primaquine and the primaquone analog tafenoquine may be future alternatives but otherwise there are few new drugs for chemoprophylaxis on the horizon [19]. Vivax malaria causes significant illness in travelers, but relapses of vivax malaria are not prevented with the current first-line chemoprophylaxis regimens [16].Exotic illnesses in the returned traveler are of concern to the physician because they often strike an otherwise young and healthy segment of the population and may carry significant morbidity and mortality if not recognized early [20]. Fever in travelers returning from the tropics may be caused not only by tropical infection but also by travel associated non-specific infections and cosmopolitan infective diseases [21]. The infrequency with which these diseases are encountered demands a systematic approach to history, a physical exam, and the construction of a differential diagnosis [20]. Information about the geographic distribution, routes of transmission, and incubation periods of the pathogens allows a clinician to reduce the differential to a manageable number of the likeliest etiologies [20]. However, a reversed process namely pre-traveling counseling is more proper [22]. A travel risk assessment is an essential component of travel consultation, and is an efficient way of providing international travelers with evidence-based advice [23].

Malaria and Travel Medicine in Southeast Asia

1. Traveler and Malaria in Southeast Asia

Southeast Asia is now one of the most famous destinations for vacation of the western populations. Similar to any destination, the importance of travel medicine for the traveler should be mentioned. Malaria in the traveler during and after traveling to Southeast Asia is reported. For decades, malaria in Thailand has been largely confined to rural areas principally along the borders with Cambodia and Myanmar [24 – 25]. Due to the present rapid travel industrial growth, the effect of the traveling on the epidemiology pattern of malaria can be expected. For the foreign tourists who visited Thailand, somecases of malaria during traveling can be detected. Although the total number of cases are not high and it can reflect the necessary of the recommendation for chemoprophylxis for the travelers [26]. Since the traveling is the main business for Thailand, the informationfor the primary health prevention should be included in the promotion for tourism.Because the tourists have no immunity to many tropical diseases, which is stillprevalent in Thailand, the physicians who get the consultation from the foreign tourists should be aware for these diseases. Indeed, there are some sporadic cases of malaria in the tourists returning from Southeast Asia to their hometown [27 – 28]. According to an analysis of imported case of malaria in Australia, malaria is most commonly acquired in Papua New Guinea and Southeast Asia [29]. The median times to diagnosis after return to Australia for *P. falciparum* and *P. vivax* infections are 1 and 9 weeks respectively [29]. Travelers returning from Papua New Guinea are eight times more likely to relapse after primaquine treatment compared to travelers with *P. vivax* malaria acquired elsewhere [30]. The primary care physician should have a high index of suspicion for malaria in the traveler returning from the tropics [31].

2. Migrant and Malaria in Southeast Asia

In Thailand, the migrant workers from the nearby countries, the infections were firstly detected in Thailand without previous history of diagnosis or treatment in their hometown is an important group of imported malarial cases. Of interest, these cases comprise of a large proportion of registry malaria cases. Apart from some usually mentioned problems in malaria control in Thailand as technical, operational and social obstacles, a possible cause of this phenomenon may be due to the imported cases of malaria via the migrants. Presently, thousands of migrant workers live in Thailand, working as the laborers. A number of these workers are illegal. Also, these workers are usually a carrier of many diseases including to malaria [32]. Considering the migrant, residence located in the forest increased the risk of malaria infection [33].Fortunately, after the recent national policy for control of migrant workers, the annual incidence of malaria was decrease. Therefore, control and screening program for these migrant workers are necessary.

3. Malaria and Refugee

In the past two decades, refugee emerged from several countries of Southeast Asia due to warfare. It is worth to mention to the malarial problem in this type of traveling. The high frequency of infectious diseases in refugees compared with the new community leads to a recommendation for continuing medical examinations and treatment for new refugees [34]. The refugees' infectious medical problems are generally common rather than exotic, although unusual diagnoses must occasionally be considered. If diagnosed, they are generally amenable to treatment [35]. They pose little risk to the public health, and the little danger that they do represent can largely be obviated by attention to principles of infection control, personal hygiene, and public sanitation [35]. In 1980, Guerrero et al performed a study to assess the prevalence of malaria among Indochinese refugees in USA [36]. According to this study, the malaria infection rate was at least 1.7% based on blood smear examination but might be as high as 45% based on serologic examinations [36]. The results of this study when combined with malaria surveillance indicate that the likelihood of introduced malaria in the United States from the Indochinese refugees is low [36].

Specific Recommendation for the Traveler on Malaria in Southeast Asia

Primary prevention for malaria is recommended for the travelers who plan to have a traveling in Southeast Asia. The malarial risk for each specific area is listed in Table 1 [37]. More details for primary prevention of malaria can be seen in the chapter of mosquito prevention.

Table 1. The malarial risk for each specific area in Southeast Asia.

Risk level	Areas
High	Myanmar, Laos, Cambodia, Eastern Timor
Average	Malaysia, the Philipines, Thailand, Vietnam
Low	Singapore, Brunei Darussalam, capitals and big cities of all countries

References

[1] Chareonviriyaphap T, Bangs MJ, Ratanatham S. Status of malaria in Thailand. *Southeast Asian J Trop Med Public Health* 2000; 31: 225-237.

[2] Thimasarn K, Jatapadma S, Vijaykadga S et al. Epidemiology of Malaria in Thailand. *J Travel Med* 1995; 2:59-65.

[3] Sutherst RW. Global change and human vulnerability to vector-borne diseases. *Clin Microbiol Rev*. 2004;17:136-73.

[4] Wiwanitkit V. Amazing Thailand Year 1998-1999 Tourist's health concepts. *Chula Med J* 1998: 47: 975-984.

[5] DeHart RL. Health issues of air travel. *Annu Rev Public Health*. 2003;24:133-51.

[6] Pinheiro FP, Corber SJ. Global situation of dengue and dengue haemorrhagic fever, and its emergence in the Americas. *World. Health. Stat. Q*. 1997; 50: 161- 9.

[7] Haas W, Krause G, Marcus U, Stark K, Ammon A, Burger R. Emerging infectious diseases". Dengue-fever, West-Nile-fever, SARS, avian influenza, HIV. *Internist* (Berl). 2004; 45: 684-92.

[8] Badiaga S, Barrau K, Brouqui P, Durant J, Malvy D, Janbon F, Bonnet E, Bosseray A, Sotto A, Peyramont D, Dydymski S, Cazorla C, Tolou H, Durant JP, Delmont J; Infectio-Sud Group. Imported Dengue in French University Hospitals: a 6-year survey. *J Travel Med*. 2003; 10: 286-9.

[9] Gascon J, Giner V, Vidal J, Jou JM, Mas E, Corachan M. Dengue: a re-emerging disease. A clinical and epidemiological study in 57 Spanish travelers. *Med Clin*. (Barc). 1998; 111: 583-6.

[10] Newsom EY. South Carolina's last yellow fever epidemic: Manning Simons at Port Royal, 1877. *JSC Med Assoc*. 1995; 91: 311-3.
[11] Monath TP. Facing up to re-emergence of urban yellow fever. *Lancet*. 1999; 353: 1541.
[12] Tomori O. Yellow fever: the recurring plague. *Crit Rev Clin Lab Sci*. 2004; 41: 391-427.
[13] WHO. Yellow fever vaccine. Available at http://www.who.int/vaccines/en/yellowfever.shtml Van Laethem Y. Vaccinations for the traveler. *J Pharm Belg* 2002; 57: 130-4
[14] Khan AS, Qureshi F, Shah AH, Malik SA. Spectrum of malaria in Hajj pilgrims in the year 2000. *J Ayub Med Coll Abbottabad*. 2002;14:19-21.b
[15] Chen LH, Wilson ME, Schlagenhauf P. Prevention of malaria in long-term travelers. *JAMA*. 2006;296:2234-44.
[16] Chiodini J. Malaria in UK travellers: assessment, prevention and treatment. *Nurs Stand*. 2006;20:49-57
[17] Petersen JE. Malaria chemoprophylaxis. *Ugeskr Laeger*. 2005;167:3984-7.
[18] Petersen JE. Malaria chemoprophylaxis: when should we use it and what are the options? *Expert Rev Anti Infect Ther*. 2004;2:119-32.
[19] Schwartz MD. Fever in the returning traveler, part one: A methodological approach to initial evaluation. Wilderness Environ Med. 2003;14:24-32.
[20] Ziegler T, Schau A, Winkler C, Funfstuck R. Fever after travel to the tropics. *Med Klin* (Munich). 2002;97:30-3.
[21] Dick L. Travel medicine: helping patients prepare for trips abroad. *Am Fam Physician*. 1998;58:383-98, 401-2.
[22] Stringer C, Chiodini J, Zuckerman J. International travel and health assessment. *Nurs Stand*. 2002;16:49-54.
[23] Thimasarn K, Jatapadma S, Vijaykadga S, Sirichaisinthop J, Wongsrichanalai C. Epidemiology of Malaria in Thailand. *J Travel Med* 1995;2:59-65.
[24] Chareonviriyaphap T, Bangs MJ, Ratanatham S. Status of malaria in Thailand. *Southeast Asian J Trop Med Public Health* 2000;31:225-37.
[25] CDC. CDC health information for travelers to Southeast Asia. Available on Http://www.cdc.gov/travel/regionalmalaria/seasia.htm. 2002.
[26] Waksman JC, Huminer D, Keller N, Pitlik SD. Delayed synchronous outbreak of Plasmodium vivax malaria in four travelers. *J Travel Med*. 1999;6:142-3.
[27] Ekvall H, Aust-Kettis A, Bjorkman A. Severe falciparum malaria among travellers to Thailand. Blood exchange and artemisinine treatment are therapeutic alternatives. *Lakartidningen*. 1997;94:1713-5.
[28] Robinson P, Jenney AW, Tachado M, Yung A, Manitta J, Taylor K, Biggs BA. Imported malaria treated in Melbourne, Australia: epidemiology and clinical features in 246 patients. *J Travel Med*. 2001;8:76-81.
[29] Elliott JH, O'Brien D, Leder K, Kitchener S, Schwartz E, Weld L, Brown GV, Kain KC, Torresi J, GeoSentinel Surveillance Network Imported Plasmodium vivax malaria: demographic and clinical features in nonimmune travelers. *J Travel Med.* 2004;11:213-7.
[30] Heck JE. Malaria. Prim Care. 1991;18:195-211.
[31] Wiwanitkit V. High prevalence of malaria in Myanmar migrant workers in a rural district near the Thailand – Myanmar border. *Scand J Infect Dis* 2002; 34: 236 – 7.

[32] Chaveepojnkamjorn W, Pichainarong N. Malaria infection among the migrant population along the Thai-Myanmar border area. *Southeast Asian J Trop Med Public Health.* 2004;35:48-52.

[33] Katsumata T, Kohno S, Yamashita K, Takeno Y, Matsunaga K, Oka R, Fujiwara T, Hara K. Health problems among Vietnamese refugees resettled in Japan. *Southeast Asian J Trop Med Public Health.* 1993;24:647-53.

[34] Dashefsky B, Teele DW. Infectious disease problems in indochinese refugees. Pediatr Ann. 1983;12:232-44.

[35] Guerrero IC, Chin W, Collins WE. A survey of malaria in Indochinese refugees arriving in the United States, 1980. Am J Trop Med Hyg. 1982;31:897-901.

[36] Travelers' Health: Regional Malaria Information. Available online at http://www.cdc.gov/travel/regionalmalaria/seasia.htm

Chapter 12

Mosquito Prevention

Abstract

Mosquito prevention is important for control of malaria and other mosquito-borne infectious diseases. In this article, the concepts based on preventive medicine for mosquito-borne infectious diseases are presented. Primary, secondary and tertiary prevention for the mosquito-borne infectious diseases are reviewed and discussed.

Overview of Preventive Medicine in Mosquito-Borne Diseases

Generally, preventive medicine covers three levels: primary, secondary and tertiary prevention [1]. Concerning primary prevention, prevention from starting of the unwanted event, infection in this case, is focused. The primary prevention can be the control of vector, immunization as well as chemophophylaxis. Concerning secondary prevention, early detection and prompt treatment is focused. Identify and treat asymptomatic persons who have already developed risk factors or preclinical infectious disease is in this step. The efficiency of preventive treatments should lead toward the goal of zero infectious cases [2]. Concerning tertiary prevention, the control of disability or sequelae, including physical, psychological as well as social items, is focused. For example, the application of the three - leveled prevention in case of filariasis is presented in Table 1

Table 1 Application of the three - leveled prevention in case of filariasis

Level of prevention	Example of activity
Primary	Insecticide spraying
Secondary	Screening test by blood smear interpretation
Tertiary	Rehabitation for elephantiasis

In order to get success in prevention and control of mosquito-borne disease, updating on the data of those diseases are necessary. Basic information is required before planning and launching of any preventive strategies. New technology should be applied for this purpose.

Recently, Roberts and Rodriguez demonstrated the value of remote sensing technology for studying mosquito-borne diseases [3]. They noted that many recent studies had also shown that it was necessary to fully define the environmental factors associated with the presence of vectors and disease transmission, and to be able to detect these environmental factors with image data [3]. Singer and de Castro mentioned that basic information required for planning of a successful preventive and control program for mosquito-borne diseases should include the data on interrelationships between macropolitical, social and economic policies, human migration, agricultural development, and disease transmission [4]. They also proposed for the useful of many spatial statistical methodologies linked to a geographical information system (GIS) to describe the patterns of human settlement in the area, the ecological transformations induced by local occupational practices, and the manner in which these factors determine gradations of mosquito-borne infections risk [4].

PRIMARY PREVENTION FOR MOSQUITO-BORNE DISEASE

Vector Control

Vector control is a basic useful primary prevention that can be applied for all mosquito-borne diseases. Since all mosquito-borne diseases are vector-borne diseases, therefore, the control of vector is rational in prevention. Historically, Mulla said that control technology in the first half of the 20th century was relatively simple, utilizing source reduction, larvivorous fish, petroleum hydrocarbon oils, and some simple synthetic and botanical materials and during the 2nd half of the 20th century, however, various classes of synthetic organic chemicals, improved petroleum oil formulations, insect growth regulators, synthetic pyrethroids, and microbial control agents were developed and employed in mosquito control and control of other disease-vectoring insects [5]. Mulla also noted that t is likely that petroleum oil formulations, insect growth regulators, and microbial control agents will provide the main thrust against vectors at least during the first quarter of the 21st century [5]. Several present methods for mosquito vector control are hereby presented.

Insecticide

Pesticides can be classified according to their use (insecticides, fungicides, herbicides or raticides) or by their chemical family (organochlorates, organophosphates, carbamates, pyrethroids, Bipyridilium compounds or inorganic salts). An insecticide is a pesticide whose purpose is to kill or to prevent the multiplication of insects [6]. Insecticides are very widely used in agriculture, as well as in people's dwellings and workplaces [6]. The use of insecticides is one of the major causal factors behind the increase in agricultural productivity in the 20th century [6]. Although insecticide poses a lot of advantage for human it, on the other hand bring several hazardous effects. Yan *et al* said that in the developing countries, there was a need to study the toxicological effects of mixtures of metals, pesticides, and organic compounds [7]. They said that the study of mixtures containing substances such as DDT (dichlorodiphenyltrichloroethane, an insecticide banned in developed nations), and mixtures containing contaminants such as fluoride (of concern only in developing countries) merit special attention [7]. Soogarun *et al* recently reported decreased serum cholinesterase levels among a sample of a rural Thai population, who were in the agricultural communities [8]. Soogarun *et al* also reported that the mean blood cholinesterase level, biomarker for insecticide exposure, in vegetable growers was significantly lower than that of the control group [9]. In additional to the main purpose in agriculture, insecticide is also applied in public health.

In mosquito control, insecticide is widely used. Mulla said that among those groups of control agents, petroleum oil formulations have endured to be used through the whole century [5]. DDT is the most widely used insecticide aiming at mosquito control. Turusov *et al* said that due to uncontrolled use for several decades, DDT, probably the best known and most useful insecticide in the world, had damaged wildlife and might have negative effects on human health [10]. They noted that even though its usd has been prohibited in most countries for ecologic considerations, mainly because of its negative impact on wildlife, it was still used in some developing countries for essential public health purposes, and it was still produced for export in at least three countries [10]. Due to its stability and its capacity to accumulate in adipose tissue, it is found in human tissues, and there is now not a single living organism on the planet that does not contain DDT [10]. Marine mammals were also reported for highly exposure to this organochlorine [11]. In 2001, Pandit et al performed an interesting study to determine organochlorine pesticide residues in sediment and fish samples collected from the east and west coasts of India [12]. They found that despite the higher quantity of consumption, DDT levels in fish in India were lower than those in temperate countries suggesting a lower accumulation in tropical fish, which could be due to rapid volatilization and degradation of these insecticides in the tropical environment [12]. They concluded that the high temperature in the tropics also enhanced the elimination rate of chemicals in fish, as the biological half-lives of semivolatile compounds such as DDT are short at high temperature.Turusov *et al* also mentioned for the possible contribution of DDT to increasing the risks for cancers at various sites and its possible role as an endocrine disruptor [10]. Organochlorine pesticides especially for DDT, the first to be used in massive fumigations to fight mosquito-borne disease, have received the most attention because of their persistence in the environment, ability to concentrate up the food chain, continued detection in the food supply and breast milk, and ability to be stored in the adipose tissue of animals and humans [13 - 14]. There is convincing experimental evidence for the carcinogenicity of DDT and of its main metabolite dichlorodiphenyldichloroethylene (DDE) [10]. Several early descriptive studies and a cohort study identified a strong positive association with cancer risk and adipose or blood levels of the organochlorine pesticide DDT and/or its metabolite DDE [14]. However, epidemiologic studies have provided contrasting or inconclusive, although prevailingly negative, results [10]. Turusov *et al* said that efficient pesticides that did not have the negative properties of DDT, together with the development of alternative methods to fight mosquito-borne, should be sought with the goal of completely banning DDT [10, 15]. Of interest, Roberts *et al* said that since the ban of DDT in the 1970s and the implementation of alternative malaria-control programs there had been a global outburst of malaria epidemics, therefore, it was recommended that the global response to burgeoning malaria rates allow for DDT residual house spraying where it was known to be effective and necessary [16]. They proposed that regulations and policies of industrialized countries and international agencies that block financial assistance to countries that use DDT for malaria control should be eliminated [16].

Another consideration for usage of insecticide in the present day is the resistance of mosquito. Roberts and Andre said that both insecticidal and behavioral effects of insecticides were important [17]. In addition, the genetic selection of insecticide resistance (whether physiological, biochemical or behavioral) in pests and disease vectors has been extensively reported worldwide [18]. Early studies of DDT showed repellent, irritant, and toxic actions that worked against vector mosquitoes [16]. Sprayed on house walls, DDT exerted powerful control over indoor transmission of mosquto-borne disease [16]. Roberts and Andre said that many field studies in Africa, India, Brazil, and Mexico provided persuasive evidence for strong behavioral avoidance of DDT by the primary vector species and this avoidance behavior, exhibited when msoquito vectors avoid insecticides by not entering or by rapidly exiting sprayed houses, should raise serious questions about the overall value of current physiological and biochemical resistance tests [17]. Roberts and Andre conclude that each insecticide chemical should be studied early before broad-scale use to define types of action against vector species by geographic area [17]. In India and Zanzibar, DDT resistance in vectors, as well as a decline in spray coverage, are probable causes of reduced effectiveness of DDT in recent decades [19]. In Thailand, vector resistance after the long use of insecticide is also mentioned [18]. Chareonviriyahpap *et al* said that the long-term intensive use of chemical pesticides to control insect pests and disease vectors was often cited as the reason behind the development of insecticide resistance in insect population [18].

Biolarvicide

In additional to the insecticide, chemical toxin, there is an attempt to use some biological toxin for controlling mosquito vectors. Biolarvicides, based on mosquitocidal toxins of certain microorganisms are highly effective against mosquito larvae at very low doses and safe to other non-target organisms [20]. There are a number of microbial agents including fungus, protozoa, virus and bacteria, which act as mosquitocidal agents [21]. However, among these agents, *Bacillus thuringiensis* var israelensis and *Bacillus sphaericus* are the most potent mosquitocidal agents [21]. *Bacillus thuringiensis* var israelensis and *Bacillus sphaericus* are gram-positive sporulating bacteria, which produce protoxin crystals during sporulation and are highly toxic to susceptible mosquito larvae when they ingest them [21]. Bhattacharya said that these bacterial agents were environmentally safe due to their host specificity, require in very low dosage, easy to prepare commercially in large-scale and are less costly [21]. Bhattacharya also noted that field trials with various formulations of *Bacillus sphaericus* and *Bacillus thuringiensis* var israelensis had demonstrated their safety and potential for controlling mosquitoes [21]. In additional to *Bacillus* spp, genetically altered *Agmenellum quadruplicatum* PR-6 is also shown to be toxic to larvae of three major genera of disease-bearing mosquitoes [22]. A fungus, *Lagenidium giganteum*, was also reported to be an effective biolarvicide [23].

Larvivourous Fish

Recently, because of concern about the effects of insecticide on the environment, increased attention is being given to the use of biological agents for controlling the vectors of human disease [24]. Biological control may encompass the use of predators, pathogens, parasites, pheromones, insect growth regulators, and other factors [24]. Larvivorous fish is a predator, natural enemy, to mosquito larvae [24]. Hwang and Chow said that since 1988, larvivorous fish, mainly *Gambusia affinis*, had been employed for controlling Aedes larvae in water containers in Taiwan [24]. In India, Sharma performed studies to assess the role of some indigenous fish of Haryana state for the biological control of mosquitoes [25]. In this study, total of 28 fish species were encountered and Sharma found that only 6 fresh water fish species *Puntius ticto*, *Colisa fasciata*, *Aplocheilus panchax*, *Rasbora daniconius*, *Chanda nama*, and *Esomus danricus* species possessed good feeding potential on mosquito larvae [25]. Haq *et al* performed a similar study in Shahjahanpur on 35 indigenous fish species. They found that 24 out of 35 fish species were found feeding on mosquito larvae of which 6 species including *Chela bacaila*, *Puntius stigma*, *Rasbora daniconius*, *Esomus danricus*, *Colisa fasciatus* and *Danio* spp, had good larvivorous potential [26]. They found that difference in the feeding capacity of fishes in the months of September and January was highly significant but there was no seasonal variation in the preference of consumption [26]. In Ethiopia, a randomized controlled trial was carried out in Assab under the auspices of the National Organization for the Control of Malaria and other Vectorborne Diseases to assess the effectiveness of an indigenous cyprinodontid fish, *Aphanius dispar*, in controlling mosquito larvae, including the local malaria vector [27]. According to this study, stocking of larvivorous fish in wells and household water storage containers was well-accepted by the participants, who were aware of the role of the fish in malaria prevention and found the fish useful in keeping their water free of other aquatic organisms [27]. According to another similar study by Fletcher *et al*, two priority areas for the assessment of biological control using larvivorous fish were identified, the port city of Assab, using the local species *Aphanius dispar*, and the Ogaden, south-eastern Ethiopia, using the local species *Oreochromis spilurus* [28].

Transgenic Mosquito

In recent years, mosquito molecular biology has been a scene of astounding achievements, namely the development of genetic transformation, characterization of inducible tissue-specific promoters, and acquirement of mosquito genome sequences [29]. The development of efficient germ-line transformation technologies for mosquitoes has increased the ability of entomologists to find, isolate and analyze genes [30]. The advantage of transgenesis is the ability to establish genetically stable, dominant-negative and overexpression phenotypes [29]. Potential applications for reducing transmission of mosquito-borne diseases by releasing genetically modified mosquitoes have been proposed, and mosquitoes are being created with such an application in mind in several laboratories [31]. Benedict and Robinson Said that the use of the sterile insect technique (SIT) provided a safe program in which production, release and mating competitiveness questions related to mass-reared genetically modified mosquitoes could be answered [31]. Presently, transgenic mosquito is applied for control of many mosquito-borne diseases especially for malaria and yellow fever [32].

Environmental Management

Environmental management is an important part in vector control since one of important contributing factors for mosquito spreading is environmental factor. Lacey and Lacey said that some of the elements of environmental management for mosquitoes in rice field, including malaria and Japanese encephalitis mosquito vectors, should include the use of intermittent irrigation; flushing of fields; use of rice cultivars that require less water; shifting of planting schedules to avoid optimal mosquito breeding conditions; relocation of communities or use of dry belt farming around them [23]. Careful siting of settlements is also a successful, but hard to perform, method prevent man-mosquito contact [32]. In houses, window and door screening are basic practice [32]. Additional anti-larval measures using enviromental management aiming at source reduction are useful [33]. Protection of wells and water reservoirs are the main anti-larval measures in house [33]. In Thailand, a highly endemic country for dengue, water storage containers, especially water jars, served as a main larval breeding habitats of *Aedes aegypti*, whereas broken cans and plastic containers are considered primary breeding sites for *Aedes alpopictus* during the dry period [34]. Water container management methods are specifically recommended for the control of dengue [35]. Using of abate sand for larvicidal purpose is also recommended [34]. Indeed, the survey of mosquito vector and container are important in surveillance for dengue infection. Aedes larval indices, container index (CI), house index (HI), and Breteau index (BI) are the important parameter in those surveillance.

Mechanical Control of Mosquito

The most basic mechanical control of mosquito is direct hand clapping on the mosquitoes. Presently, many electronic devices for mosquito clapping are produced. In addition, there are more applications by combination between mechanical machine and chemical reagent in control of mosquitoes. Ground ULV machine is a good example. Dukes et al performed a study to determine the effects of machine pressure and insecticide flow rate on the size of aerosol droplets as they relate to the Cythion label was conducted with 3 different ground ULV aerosol generators [36]. They found that an increase in flow rate required a corresponding increase in blower pressure to maintain the labeled droplet mass median diameter of 17 microns or less and droplets larger than 48 microns were frequently sampled at machine pressures less than 6 psi (41.4 kPa) [36]. They noted that machine pressures of 7-8 psi (48.3-55.2 kPa) were required for each of the 3 aerosol generators tested to consistently conform to the droplet criteria of the Cythion label at the highest labeled flow rate of 8.6 fl oz/min (254.3 ml/min) [36]. Recently, a new method for delivering microbial mosquito control agents into aquatic sites as ice granules for mosquito control was proposed [37]. A special ice-making machine were used to transform solutions containing powder formulations of *Bacillus sphaericus* into ice pellets, named IcyPearls [37]. Becker said that this new technique was demonstrated to have the following advantages over Bti sand granules: 1) the Bti ice pellets melted on the water surface and released the microbial crystals there; 2) the control agent remained inside the ice pellets during the application and were not lost by friction in the spraying equipment; and 3) the ice formulation resulted in increased swath widths, significantly reducing the cost of application [37]. In large field tests. IcyPearls have been applied at dosages of 5 and 10 kg/ha containing 400 g as well as 100, 200, and 400 g of VectoBac WDG (3,000 ITU/mg), respectively, against larvae of *Aedes vexans* [37].

Entomopathogen

Biological control agents that have been used successfully in mosquito control include several species of larvivorous fish, biolarvicide and a mermithid nematode [23]. The mermithid, an entomopathogen, has demonstrated little or no adverse effects on populations of vertebrate and invertebrate nontarget organisms [23].

Many mermithid such as *Romanomermis culicivorax* and *Strelkovimermis spiculatus* are used in control of mosquito. Achinelly and Garcia said that extended longevity with maintenance of the infectivity capacity of preparasites, are important attributes to consider *Strelkovimermis spiculatus* an effective mean of controlling a large number of culicid species between 4 and 27 degrees C [38]. In 2000, Paily and Balaraman studied susceptibility of ten species of mosquito larvae to the parasitic nematode *Romanomermis iyengari* [39]. In this study, ten species of mosquitoes from five genera were exposed to preparasites of the tropical mermithid nematode species *Romanomermis iyengari* [39]. By exposing mosquito larvae during the second instar, nematode infection was invariably lethal, the rate being highest in *Culex sitiens*followed by Culex quinquefasciatus, Aedes aegypti, Anopheles subpictus, Aedes albopictus and Armigeres subalbatus, Culex tritaeniorhynchus, Mansonia annulifera , Anopheles stephensi and Anopheles culicifacies [39]. They found that the parasitic phase of the nematode lasted 5-7 days in all the host species, yielding 1.1-3.2 parasites per II instar and 1.1-2.5 parasites per IV instar and the overall output of parasites per 100 mosquito larvae, both infected and uninfected, was highest for Aedes aegypti when mosquitoes were exposed during II instar and lowest for Mansonia annulifera exposed during IV instar [39]. In 1994, Santamarina Mijares studied the feasibility on usage of *Romanomermis culicivorax nematode* for the control of 3 mosquito species: *Anopheles albimanus*, *Culex nigripalpus* and *Uranotaenia saphirina*, in 10 natural reservoirs [40]. According to this study, increased infestation indices were observed with values ranging from 1.2 to 3.4; mortality percentages fluctuated between 70 and 97% depending on the mosquito species found in the reservoirs [40]. Santamarina Mijares found that anophelines showed more susceptibility to parasite infection; culicines showed a lower susceptibility in general and mosquito larva populations were significantly reduced in the treated reservoirs [40].

Bednet

Self-protection against mosquito bites by bednets, especially those impregnated with synthetic pyrethroids, are simple vector control method. Lindsay and Gibson said that bednets, especially nets impregnated with repellant or insecticide, were attracting increasing interest as a key intervention against mosquito-borne parasites. They said that bednets were relatively cheap and simple to use, and if arranged correctly could give protection against mosquitoes and other nocturnal biting flies [41]. Binka *et al* said that the cost-effectiveness of bednet impregnation was sufficiently attractive to make it part of a package of high priority interventions [42]. In Gambia, Aikins *et al* said that adding the cost of all mosquito nets would increase the cost-effectiveness ratios by over five times, which was an important consideration for countries with a lower coverage of mosquito nets per capita [43]. They also noted that insecticide-impregnated mosquito nets were one of the more efficient ways of reducing deaths in children under 10 years in rural Gambia [43]. In China, Zhang and Yang said that the effects of the impregnated-bednets on *Anopheles sinensis* were different, even opposite, between different investigations, however, the treated bednets caused the density of *Anopheles minimus* in houses to fall by 67.94%, and the total density in houses and cattle shelters by 67.91% [44]. Of interest, Rowland *et al* said that there was no difference in malaria prevalence between buyers and non-buyers at the time of net sales [45].

In additional to insecticide-treated bednet, there are also other insecticide-treated materials for mosquito control. Rowland *et al* said that insecticide-treated mosquito nets provided excellent protection against malaria; however, they had a number of shortcomings that were particularly evident in politically unstable countries or countries at war: not everyone at risk can necessarily afford a net, nets might be difficult to obtain or import, nets might not be suitable for migrants or refugees sleeping under tents or plastic shelter [46]. Rowland *et al* said that there was a need to develop cheaper, locally appropriate alternatives for the most impoverished and for victims of complex emergencies [46]. Concerning other insecticide-treated materials, chaddars and top-sheets are the good example. Rowland *et al* said that permethrin-treated top-sheets and blankets should provide appropriate and effective protection from malaria in complex emergencies [46]. They also noted that treated chaddars and top-sheets should offer a satisfactory solution for the most vulnerable who cannot afford treated nets in Islamic and non-Islamic countries in Asia [46]. Kroeger *et al* noted that the protective efficacy of insecticide-treated materials varied according to the coverage achieved: protective efficacy was 68% in communities with an average insecticide-treated material coverage of 50%; 31% in communities with an insecticide-treated material coverage of 16-30%; and no protective efficacy in communities with insecticide-treated material coverage below 16%, in Latin America [47].

Mosquito Coils and Repellents

Burning mosquito coils indoors generates smoke that can control mosquitoes effectively [48 – 49]. This practice is currently used in numerous households in Asia, Africa, and South America [49].Official guidelines commonly advise travelers to burn mosquito coils as one means of preventing malaria [48]. However, Lawrance and Croft said that there was no evidence that burning insecticide-containing mosquito coils prevents malaria acquisition, however,.there was consistent evidence that burning coils inhibits nuisance biting by various mosquito species [48]. They also suggested that potential harmful effects of coil smoke on human users should be investigated [48]. Liu *et al* said that the smoke might contain pollutants of health concern [49]. Liu *et al* conducted a to characterize the emissions from four common brands of mosquito coils using mass balance equations to determine emission rates of fine particles (particulate matter < 2.5 microm in diameter; PM(2.5)), polycyclic aromatic hydrocarbons (PAHs), aldehydes, and ketones [49]. According to this study, they identified a large suite of volatile organic compounds, including carcinogens and suspected carcinogens, in the coil smoke [49]. They suggested that exposure to the smoke of mosquito coils could pose significant acute and chronic health risks [49].

In additional to mosquito coils, repellent is another common material for mosquito prevention. Many repellents with insecticide compositions are produced and within use at present. Of interest, the effect of spraying of in-house repellents depends on the surface coverage of the house. Zhang and Yang performed a study on this topic [44]. According to this study, on walls built with cement and covered with a thin layer of lime on which deltamethrin at a dosage of 0.025 g/m2 was sprayed, 100% of the mosquitos were stricken down within 3 days, 80% at the 15th day, 50% at the 20th day while the residual effectiveness on the bamboo and wood walls was good and could last for over 40 days, but on the mud walls a mortality of only 40% on the spraying day was observed, indicating that deltamethrin was not suitable for this purpose [44]. In addition, deltamethrin spraying reduced total caught mosquitos within 30 days, but there was no difference between the effects of deltamethrin and DDT at the 60th day [44]. Presently, there are several attempts to develop natural product – based topical repellent for mosquito prevention. Lemongrass oil is a good example for the natural topical repellent. In 2002, Oyedele *et al* evaluated ointment and cream formulations of lemongrass oil in different classes of base and the oil in liquid paraffin solution for mosquito repellency in a topical application [50]. They found that the oil demonstrated efficacy from the different bases in the order of hydrophilic base, emulsion base and oleaginous base, respectively [50]. Some topical repellents are used for a long time by local population in the endemic area of mosquito-borne infectious diseases. Thanaka (*Limonia acidissima*) and deet (di-methyl benzamide) mixture as a mosquito repellent for use by Karen women who live in Thai-Myanmar borber, the highly endemic area of malaria, are good examples for those natural traditional mosquito repellents [51].

Ovitrap

Indeed, the greatest advantage of the ovitrap is the collection of adult female mosquitoes, negating the need to rear larvae for identification and providing a faster, more direct measure of the effectiveness of ovipositional attractants than egg counts [52]. For an application, the lethal ovitrap is designed to kill mosuqito via an insecticide-treated ovistrip (impregnated with deltamethrin) [53]. Ritchie *et al* noted that demonstrated that sticky ovitraps, being adulticidal, had potential as a supplementary control measure, especially for quarantine programs designed to prevent the import and export of container-breeding vector mosquitoes at sea- and airports [53]. In 2003, Perich *et al* performed a field evaluation of a lethal ovitrap against dengue vectors in Brazil [52]. They proposed for sustained impact of lethal ovitraps on dengue vector population densities in housing conditions [52]

Chemoprophylaxis

Chemoprophylaxis is an important primary prevention in malaria. Leonard *et al* said that chemoprophylaxis was most often necessary, adapted to the possibility of chloroquine resistant *Plasmodium falciparum*, to the length or conditions of travel, and to the traveler's antecedents and age [54]. They noted that chemoprophylaxis had to be continued after coming back, for a duration depending on the drug used [54].Touze *et al* said that drug prophylaxis had been recommended using a combination of 100 mg of chloroquine and 200 mg of proguanil chlorhydrate (CQ + PG) [56]. In addition, a new policy was implemented especially in countries where cycloguanil-resistant *Plasmodium falciparum* incidence rate is increasing [56]. Touze *et al* noted that the new chemoprophylactic regimen called for a personal prescription of mefloquine and doxycycline monohydrate was used in case of mefloquine contra-indication or intolerance [56]. Bouchaud *et al* noted that chemoprophylaxis by chloroquine-proguanil, mefloquine or, less frequently cyclines, was efficacious but poor compliance and frequent adverse events limits its interest [55]. However, Leonard *et al* said that no prophylaxis was 100% effective, and the appearance of fever during the travel or two to three months after return requires medical advice [54]. Bouchaud *et al* noted that no regimen was totally effective and malaria should be considered in any traveler coming back from an endemic area with fever, even still receiving an appropriate prophylaxis [55]. In some circumstances, it is necessary to prescribe a stand-by emergency treatment, if no quick medical advice is possible [54]. In addition, Leonard *et al* noted that special concern about chemoprophylaxis in pregnant woman was necessary, due to potential severity of malaria [54]. Cot and Doleron said that current recommendations called for the use of a sulfadoxine-pyrimethamine twice or three times during pregnancy in antenatal clinics and this combination was more effective as a result of strong resistance of parasites to chloroquine [57]. They noted that high cost and possible adverse effects in pregnant women prohibited routine use of mefloquine in developing countries [57]. They also proposed that integration of malaria prophylaxis into antenatal care services with nutrition and immunization measures should enhance the overall efficacy of prevention in outlying clinical facilities [57].

Vaccination

Vaccination is available for some tropical mosquito-borne diseases, especially for Japanese encephalitis virus infection and yellow fever. The details of the vaccination in Japanese encephalitis and yellow fever are presented in the previous corresponding chapters. There are also several attempts to develop new vaccine for the other mosquito-borne diseases such as malaria, dengue infection and West Nile virus infection.

Zooprophylaxis

Zooprophylaxis is the diversion of disease carrying insects from humans to animals and refers to the control of vector-borne diseases by attracting vectors to domestic animals in which the pathogen cannot amplify, a dead-end host. Zooprophylaxis is mentioned for primary prevention for many mosquito-borne infectious diseases. Zooprophylaxis has been proposed as a means for malaria control since the onset of the previous century to the present day [58]. A good example of zooprophylaxis is using cattle as zooprophylaxis of malaria, the human malarial parasite has a closed transmission cycle between humans and mosquitoes, and hence cattle can serve as a dead-end host. Bogh *et al* said that the World Health

Organization had recommended the use of cattle for zooprophylaxis as a protective measure against malaria since 1982, however, concern had been raised about this practice, since some studies had shown that the presence of cattle may instead increase malaria prevalence [59]. In 2002, Bogh *et al* performed an interesting study to investigate the effect of passive zooprophylaxis on malaria in an area of moderate seasonal transmission in the Gambia, West Africa [59]. They found that although the presence of cattle appeared to be protective against high parasitaemia, cattle were also associated with greater wealth of the children's families and conditional logistic regression analysis showed that the decreased risk of high parasitaemia in the group with cattle present was an artefact associated with the higher general wealth of the cattle owners [59]. Bogh *et al* concluded that zooprophylaxis was not an effective intervention method against malaria [59]. In 2003, Saul said that as the number of animals increases, improved availability of blood meals might increase mosquito survival, thereby countering the impact of diverting feeds [60].Sual used computer simulation to examine the effects of animals on the transmission of human diseases by mosquitoes [60]. Sual used three scenarios model as a) endemic transmission, where the animals cannot be infected, b) epidemic transmission, where the animals cannot be infected but humans remain susceptible and c) epidemic disease, where both humans and animals can be infected, but develop sterile immunity [60]. Saul found that changing animal numbers and accessibility had little impact for endemic and epidemic mosquito-borne infectious disease with significant searching-associated vector mortality and changing the accessibility of the humans had a much greater effect while the most critical factor was the proximity of the animals to the mosquito breeding sites for diseases with an animal amplification cycle [60]

Saul concluded that zooprophylaxis might be ineffective with realistic values of searching-associated vector mortality rates, however, use of animals as bait to attract mosquitoes to insecticide was predicted to be a promising strategy [60]. Recently, Kawaguchi *et al* said that combining zooprophylaxis and insecticide spraying might be an effective malaria-control strategy limiting the development of insecticide resistance in vector mosquitoes [61].

Control of Amplifying Host

Amplifying host plays important roles in transmission of many mosquito-borne infectious diseases. Japanese encephalitis virus infection is a good example. An important amplifying host for Japanese encephalitis virus is pig. Protection of pigs against mosquito-borne Japanese encephalitis virus by immunization with a live attenuated vaccine is recommended. Sasaki *et al* found that the vaccinated pigs developed circulating antibodies to Japanese encephalitis virus and after challenge they did not develop viremia detectable by inoculation of their serum in suckling mice and they were also unable to transmit virus to mosquitoes fed on their skin [62]. In contrast, unvaccinated pigs, whether challenged by injection or by mosquito bites, developed viremia and did transmit virus to mosquitoes, which were allowed to bite them [62]. Concerning West Nile virus infection, bird is mentioned as an important amplifying host. Control of bird is necessary in this case. There are several attempts to develop avian West Nile virus vaccine. Recently, Turell *et al* evaluated a DNA vaccine for West Nile virus to determine whether its use could protect fish crows (*Corvus ossifragus*) from fatal West Nile virus infection [63]. In this study, captured adult crows were given 0.5 mg of the DNA vaccine either orally or by intramuscular (IM) inoculation; control crows were inoculated or orally exposed to a placebo [63]. Turell *et al* found that although oral administration of a single DNA vaccine dose failed to elicit an immune response or protect crows from West Nile virus infection, IM administration of a single dose prevented death and was associated with reduced viremia [63]. In severe outbreak, an important consideration in control of amplifying host is destroyed the suspected infected animals in the outbreak area.

SECONDARY PREVENTION FOR MOSQUITO-BORNE DISEASE

Secondary prevention for mosquito-borne disease included early diagnosis and prompt treatment of diseases as previously mentioned. Kager said that malaria control was based on four principles: early diagnosis and treatment; selective and sustainable preventive measures, including vector control; detection, containment and prevention of epidemics, and building up of local capacity [64]. Bosman *et al* said that early diagnosis and prompt treatment could reduce malaria mortality, but there was still low investment on safe and effective modalities of care delivery at the periphery, where most of the malaria burden existed [65]. They noted that in most countries forecasting, early detection and containment of malaria epidemics was deficient, and there was separation between the research and control communities, particularly in Africa [65].In 1992 the new Global Malaria Control Strategy adopted by Malaria Summit at Amsterdam says the primary objective is early diagnosis and treatment to prevent malaria death [66]. Concerning dengue infection, Rodriguez-Tan and Weir said that once a person is infected, the key to survival was early diagnosis and appropriate treatment for the severe, life-threatening complications of dengue hemorrhagic fever and dengue shock syndrome [67]. Guzman and Kouri G said that an appropriate rapid, early and accessible diagnostic method useful both for epidemiological surveillance and clinical diagnosis was still needed [68]. In 1996, Ramaiah *et al* studied knowledge and beliefs about transmission, prevention and control of lymphatic filariasis in rural areas of south India [69]. They said that health education campaigns aimed at highlighting the role of mosquitoes in transmission and the importance of early diagnosis could help people in taking personal protection measures and seeking appropriate treatment [69]. Indeed, the delay in visiting the physician is an important factor contributing to poor outcome of many mosquito-borne infectious diseases.

TERTIARY PREVENTION FOR MOSQUITO-BORNE DISEASE

Rehabilitation is important tertiary prevention for all mosquito-borne infectious diseases. Physical, psychological and social rehabilitation should be concerned. Lymphatic filiasis is the most common mosquito-borne infectious disease that can lead permanent disability, elephantiasis. Although the lymphatic filariasis itself is rarely fatal, the disability caused by the swollen extremities, the acute attacks of adenolymphangitis and the consequent sufferings of those afflicted are considerable [70]. Recently, Suma *et al* used semi-structured interviews, in southern India, to assess the perceptions, practices and socio-psychological problems of 127 patients with brugian filariasis [70]. They found that depression and loss of job opportunities were common in the study population [70]. Suma *et al* said that awareness of these factors would be of help in planning suitable disability-management packages, including the rehabilitation of those who found it difficult to carry on with their existing jobs because of the severity of their disease [70]. Babu and Nayak performed another interesting study to determine the economic loss in terms of treatment costs and loss of productive time because of acute episodes of adenolymphangitis (ADL) caused by lymphatic filariasis (LF) in a rural population of coastal Orissa, India [71]. According to this study, many patients were unable to attend to any economic activity [71]. The mean number of hours spent on economic or domestic activities was significantly lower among patients comparing to controls and disease status and sex had significant influence on total absenteeism from gainful employment; and similarly, age, family type and disease status influenced total domestic work hours among women [71]. Babu and Nayak concluded that there was the extent of the economic burden caused by acute lymphatic filariasis [71]. Therefore, rehabilitation for elephantiasis is very important.

References

[1] Fitzgerald MA. Primary, Secondary, and Tertiary Prevention: Important in Certification and Practice. Available at http://www.fhea.com/CertificationCols/level_prevention.htm

[2] Le Mire J, Arnulf L, Guibert P. Malaria: control strategies, chemoprophylaxis, diagnosis, and treatment. *Clin Occup Environ Med.* 2004; 4: 143-65.

[3] Roberts DR, Rodriguez MH. The environment, remote sensing, and malaria control. *Ann N Y Acad Sci.* 1994; 740: 396-402.

[4] Singer BH, de Castro MC. Agricultural colonization and malaria on the Amazon frontier. *Ann N Y Acad Sci.* 2001; 954:184-222.

[5] Mulla MS. Mosquito control then, now, and in the future. J. Am. Mosq. *Control. Assoc.* 1994; 10:574-84.

[6] Insecticide. Available at http://en.wikipedia.org/wiki/Insecticide

[7] Yan ez L, Ortiz D, Calderon J, Batres L, Carrizales L, Mejia J, Martinez L, Garcia-Nieto E, Diaz-Barriga F. Overview of human health and chemical mixtures: problems facing developing countries. *Environ. Health Perspect.* 2002; 110 Suppl 6: 901-9.

[8] Soogarun S, Wiwanitkit V, Suyaphan A, Suwansaksri J, Pathompattama N. Decreased serum cholinesterase levels among a sample of a rural Thai population. *MedGenMed.* 2003; 5: 30

[9] Soogarun S, Wiwanitkit V, Suwansaksri J. Report on blood cholinesterase among vegetable growers. *Southeast Asian J Trop Med Public Health.* 2003; 34: 687-9.

[10] Turusov V, Rakitsky V, Tomatis L. Dichlorodiphenyltrichloroethane (DDT): ubiquity, persistence, and risks. *Environ Health Perspect.* 2002; 110: 125-8.

[11] Troisi GM, Haraguchi K, Kaydoo DS, Nyman M, Aguilar A, Borrell A, Siebert U, Mason CF. Bioaccumulation of polychlorinated biphenyls (PCBs) and dichlorodiphenylethane (DDE) methyl sulfones in tissues of seal and dolphin morbillivirus epizootic victims. *J Toxicol Environ Health A.* 2001; 62: 1-8.

[12] Pandit GG, Rao AM, Jha SK, Krishnamoorthy TM, Kale SP, Raghu K, Murthy NB. Monitoring of organochlorine pesticide residues in the Indian marine environment. *Chemosphere.* 2001; 44: 301-5.

[13] Ferrer A. Pesticide poisoning. *An. Sist. Sanit. Navar. Suppl* 2003; 1: 155-71.

[14] Snedeker SM. Pesticides and breast cancer risk: a review of DDT, DDE, and dieldrin. *Environ Health Perspect*. 2001; 109 Suppl 1: 35-47.

[15] Curtis CF, Lines JD. Should DDT be banned by international treaty? *Parasitol Today*. 2000; 16:119-21.

[16] Roberts DR, Manguin S, Mouchet J. DDT house spraying and re-emerging malaria. *Lancet*. 2000; 356: 330-2.

[17] Roberts DR, Andre RG. Insecticide resistance issues in vector-borne disease control. *Am J Trop Med Hyg*. 1994; 50(6 Suppl): 21-34.

[18] Chareonviriyahpap T, Aum-aung B, Ratanatham S. Current insecticide resistance patterns in mosquito vectors in Thailand. *Southeast Asian J Trop Med Public Health*. 1999; 30: 184-94.

[19] Curtis CF. Should the use of DDT be revived for malaria vector control? *Biomedica*. 2002; 22: 455-61.

[20] Mittal PK. Biolarvicides in vector control: challenges and prospects. *J Vector Borne Dis*. 2003; 40: 20-32.

[21] Bhattacharya PR. Microbial control of mosquitoes with special emphasis on bacterial control. *Indian J Malariol*. 1998; 35: 206-24.

[22] Murphy RC, Stevens SE Jr. Development of a cyanobacterial biolarvicide. *Mem Inst Oswaldo Cruz*. 1995; 90: 109-13.

[23] Lacey LA, Lacey CM. The medical importance of riceland mosquitoes and their control using alternatives to chemical insecticides. J Am Mosq Control Assoc. Suppl. 1990; 2: 1-93.

[24] Hwang JS, Chow CY. A review of larvivorous fish. *Gaoxiong Yi Xue Ke Xue Za Zhi*. 1990; 6: 325-9.

[25] Sharma SN. Larvivorous capacity of some indigenous fish of Haryana state. *J. Commun Dis*. 1994; 26: 116-9.

[26] Haq S, Prasad H, Prasad RN, Sharma T. Availability and utility of local fishes of Shahjahanpur for mosquito control. *Indian J Malariol*. 1993; 30: 1-8.

[27] Fletcher M, Teklehaimanot A, Yemane G. Control of mosquito larvae in the port city of Assab by an indigenous larvivorous fish, Aphanius dispar. *Acta Trop*. 1992; 52:155-66.

[28] Fletcher M, Teklehaimanot A, Yemane G, Kassahun A, Kidane G, Beyene Y. Prospects for the use of larvivorous fish for malaria control in Ethiopia: search for indigenous species and evaluation of their feeding capacity for mosquito larvae. *J Trop Med Hyg*. 1993; 96: 12-21.

[29] Shin SW, Kokoza VA, Raikhel AS. Transgenesis and reverse genetics of mosquito innate immunity. *J Exp Biol*. 2003; 206(Pt 21): 3835-43.

[30] O'Brochta DA, Sethuraman N, Wilson R, Hice RH, Pinkerton AC, Levesque CS, Bideshi DK, Jasinskiene N, Coates CJ, James AA, Lehane MJ, Atkinson PW. Gene vector and transposable element behavior in mosquitoes. *J Exp Biol*. 2003; 206(Pt 21): 3823-34.

[31] Benedict MQ, Robinson AS. The first releases of transgenic mosquitoes: an argument for the sterile insect technique. *Trends Parasitol*. 2003; 19: 349-55.

[32] Christophides GK. Transgenic mosquitoes and malaria transmission. *Cell Microbiol*. 2005; 7: 325-33.

[33] Goriup S. Analysis of available measures for malaria control in Africa south of the Sahara. *Trans R Soc Trop Med Hyg*. 1989; 83 Suppl: 81-3.

[34] Chareonviriyaphap T, Akratanakul P, Nettanomsak S, Huntamai S. Larval habitats and distribution patterns of Aedes aegypti (Linnaeus) and Aedes albopictus (Skuse), in Thailand. *Southeast Asian J Trop Med Public Health.* 2003; 34: 529-35.

[35] Yap HH, Chong NL, Foo AE, Lee CY. Dengue vector control: present status and future prospects. *Gaoxiong Yi Xue Ke Xue Za Zhi.* 1994; 10 Suppl: S102-8.

[36] Dukes JC, Hallmon CF, Shaffer KR, Hester PG. Effects of pressure and flow rate on Cythion droplet size produced by three different ground ULV aerosol generators. *J Am Mosq Control Assoc.* 1990; 6: 279-82

[37] Becker N. Ice granules containing endotoxins of microbial agents for the control of mosquito larvae--a new application technique. *J Am Mosq Control Assoc.* 2003; 19, 63-6.

[38] Achinelly MF, Garcia JJ. Effect of temperature on longevity and infection with the nematode Strelkovimermis spiculatus (Nemata: Mermithidae), a parasite of mosquitoes. *Rev Biol Trop.* 2003; 51: 753-7.

[39] Paily KP, Balaraman K. Susceptibility of ten species of mosquito larvae to the parasitic nematode Romanomermis iyengari and its development. *Med Vet Entomol.* 2000; 14: 426-9.

[40] Santamarina Mijares A. Application of a mermithid nematode for the control of mosquito larvae in natural conditions. *Rev Cubana Med Trop.* 1994; 46: 115-9.

[41] Lindsay SW, Gibson ME. Bednets revisited- old idea, new angle. *Parasitol Today.* 1998; 4: 270-2.

[42] Binka FN, Mensah OA, Mills A. The cost-effectiveness of permethrin impregnated bednets in preventing child mortality in Kassena-Nankana district of Northern Ghana. *Health Policy.* 1997; 41: 229-39.

[43] Aikins MK, Fox-Rushby J, D'Alessandro U, Langerock P, Cham K, New L, Bennett S, Greenwood B, Mills A. The Gambian National Impregnated Bednet Programme: costs, consequences and net cost-effectiveness. *Soc Sci Med.* 1998; 46:181-91.

[44] Zhang Z, Yang C. Application of deltamethrin-impregnated bednets for mosquito and malaria control in Yunnan, China. *Southeast Asian J Trop Med Public. Health.* 1996; 27: 367-71.

[45] Rowland M, Webster J, Saleh P, Chandramohan D, Freeman T, Pearcy B, Durrani N, Rab A, Mohammed N. Prevention of malaria in Afghanistan through social marketing of insecticide-treated nets: evaluation of coverage and effectiveness by cross-sectional surveys and passive surveillance. *Trop Med Int Health.* 2002; 7: 813-22.

[46] Rowland M, Durrani N, Hewitt S, Mohammed N, Bouma M, Carneiro I, Rozendaal J, Schapira A. Permethrin-treated chaddars and top-sheets: appropriate technology for protection against malaria in Afghanistan and other complex emergencies. *Trans R Soc Trop Med Hyg.* 1999; 93: 465-72.

[47] Kroeger A, Gonzalez M, Ordonez-Gonzalez J. Insecticide-treated materials for malaria control in Latin America: to use or not to use? *Trans. R Soc Trop Med. Hyg.* 1999; 93: 565-70.

[48] Lawrance CE, Croft AM. Do mosquito coils prevent malaria? A systematic review of trials. *J Travel Med.* 2004;11:92-6.

[49] Liu W, Zhang J, Hashim JH, Jalaludin J, Hashim Z, Goldstein BD. Mosquito coil emissions and health implications. *Environ. Health Perspect.* 2003; 111: 1454-60.

[50] Oyedele AO, Gbolade AA, Sosan MB, Adewoyin FB, Soyelu OL, Orafidiya OO. Formulation of an effective mosquito-repellent topical product from lemongrass oil. *Phytomedicine*. 2002; 9: 259-62.
[51] Lindsay SW, Ewald JA, Samung Y, Apiwathnasorn C, Nosten F. Thanaka (Limonia acidissima) and deet (di-methyl benzamide) mixture as a mosquito repellent for use by Karen women. *Med Vet Entomol*. 1998; 12: 295-301.
[52] Perich MJ, Kardec A, Braga IA, Portal IF, Burge R, Zeichner BC, Brogdon WA, Wirtz RA. Field evaluation of a lethal ovitrap against dengue vectors in Brazil. *Med Vet Entomol*. 2003; 17: 205-10.
[53] Ritchie SA, Long S, Hart A, Webb CE, Russell RC. An adulticidal sticky ovitrap for sampling container-breeding mosquitoes. *J Am Mosq Control Assoc*. 2003; 19: 235-42.
[54] Leonard P, Moutschen M, Demonty J. Prevention of malaria in the adult. *Rev Med Liege*. 2003; 58: 382-7.
[55] Bouchaud O, Longuet C, Coulaud JP. Malaria prophylaxis. Rev Prat. 1998; 48: 279-86.
[56] Touze JE, Paule P, Baudon D, Boutin JP. Malaria prophylaxis in the French armed forces: evolution of concepts. *Med Trop* (Mars). 2001; 61: 79-82.
[57] Cot M, Deloron P. Malaria during pregnancy: consequences and interventional perspectives. *Med Trop* (Mars). 2003; 63: 369-80.
[58] Bettini S, Romi R. Zooprophylaxis: old and new problems. *Parassitologia*. 1998; 4: 423-30.
[59] Bogh C, Clarke SE, Walraven GE, Lindsay SW. Zooprophylaxis, artefact or reality? A paired-cohort study of the effect of passive zooprophylaxis on malaria in The Gambia. *Trans R Soc Trop Med Hyg*. 2002; 96: 593-6.
[60] Saul A. Zooprophylaxis or zoopotentiation: the outcome of introducing animals on vector transmission is highly dependent on the mosquito mortality while searching. *Malar J*. 2003; 2: 32.
[61] Kawaguchi I, Sasaki A, Mogi M. Combining zooprophylaxis and insecticide spraying: a malaria-control strategy limiting the development of insecticide resistance in vector mosquitoes. *Proc R Soc Lond B Biol Sci*. 2004; 271: 301-9.
[62] Sasaki O, Karoji Y, Kuroda A, Karaki T, Takenokuma K, Maeda O. Protection of pigs against mosquito-borne Japanese encephalitis virus by immunization with a live attenuated vaccine. *Antiviral Res*. 1982; 2: 355-60.
[63] Turell MJ, Bunning M, Ludwig GV, Ortman B, Chang J, Speaker T, Spielman A, McLean R, Komar N, Gates R, McNamara T, Creekmore T, Farley L, Mitchell CJ. DNA vaccine for West Nile virus infection in fish crows (Corvus ossifragus). *Emerg Infect Dis*. 2003; 9: 1077-81.
[64] Kager PA. Malaria control: constraints and opportunities. *Trop Med Int Health*. 2002; 7: 1042-6.
[65] Bosman A, Kassankogno Y, Kondrachine AV. Implementation of malaria control. *Parassitologia*. 1999; 41: 391-3.
[66] Kaneko A. Malaria on the global agenda: control and chemotherapy of malaria in Vanuatu. *Rinsho Byori*. 1998; 46: 637-44.
[67] Rodriguez-Tan RS, Weir MR. Dengue: a review. *Tex Med*. 94, 53-9 (1998)
[68] Guzman MG, Kouri G. Dengue diagnosis, advances and challenges. *Int J Infect Dis*. 2004; 8: 69-80.

[69] Ramaiah KD, Kumar KN, Ramu K. Knowledge and beliefs about transmission, prevention and control of lymphatic filariasis in rural areas of south India. *Trop Med Int Health.* 1996; 1: 433-8.

[70] Suma TK, Shenoy RK, Kumaraswami V. A qualitative study of the perceptions, practices and socio-psychological suffering related to chronic brugian filariasis in Kerala, southern India. *Ann Trop Med Parasitol.* 2003; 97: 839-45.

[71] Babu BV, Nayak AN. Treatment costs and work time loss due to episodic adenolymphangitis in lymphatic filariasis patients in rural communities of Orissa, India. *Trop Med Int Health.* 2003; 8: 1102-9.

Chapter 13

BIOCHEMOINFORMATICS TECHNOLOGY AND ANTIMALRIAL DRUG

ABSTRACT

Biochemoinformatics is a new science that can lead several advantages in medicine. New drug development can be easily performed with the new advancements in bioinformatics. Advanced biochemoinformatics technologies for drug search can be applied for new antimalarial drug search.

APPLICATION OF BIOCHEMOINFORMATICS FOR DRUG SEARCH

A. Brief History

Clinical bioinformatics provides biological and medical information to allow for individualized healthcare [1 – 2]. In the past 10 years, the field of bioinformatics has been characterized by the mapping of many genomes [1]. These efforts have stimulated explosive development of novel bioinformatics and experimental approaches to predict the functions and metabolic role of the new proteins [1]. The main application of the work is to search, validate, and prioritize new targets for designing a new generation of drugs [1]. Proteomics strategy tools usually focus on similarity searches, structure prediction, and protein modeling [2]. In clinical bioinformatics, the proteomic data only have meaning if they are integrated with clinical data. In pharmacogenomics, clinical bioinformatics includes elaborate studies of bioinformatics tools and various facets of proteomics related to drug target identification and clinical validation [2]. In the genome era upon us, researchers want rapid, easy-to-use, reliable tools for functional characterisation of newly determined sequences [3]. For the pharmaceutical industry in particular, the bioinformatics harbors an information-rich nugget, ripe with potential drug targets and possible new avenues for the development of therapeutic agents [3].

B. Bioinformatics and Drug search

Bioinformatics can be applied for new drug search. Advances in genomics, proteomics, and structural genomics have identified a large number of protein targets [4]. Virtual screening has gained popularity in identifying drug leads by computationally screening large numbers of chemicals against experimentally determined protein targets [4]. Bioinformatics is widely applied for new antibiotic search. Current research in bioinformatics relating to new antibiotic drug search can be classified into: (i) genomics--sequencing and comparative study of genomes to identify gene and genome functionality, (ii) proteomics--identification and characterization of protein related properties and reconstruction of metabolic and regulatory pathways, (iii) cell visualization and simulation to study and model cell behavior, and (iv) application to the development of drugs and anti-microbial agents [5].

For genomics, comparative genomics technique can help identification of the common sequence within the genome of human and microorganism. This can help identify the possible toxicity of the new drug. For example, Wiwanitkit performed a database search to find the recorded complete genes with complete sequences of *Mycobacterium leprae* and studied their homology to human genomes by BLAST method [6]. From a total of 35 genes, the potential candidates for further target-based drug development were identified [6]. Functional genomics can also be applied for new drug search. Functional genomics can be defined as the search for the physiological role of a gene for which only its primary sequence is known [7]. One example of a successful functional genomics adventure is the search for the natural ligands of orphan G protein-coupled receptors (GPCRs) [7]. GPCRs are proteins containing 7 hydrophobic domains that are the recognition sites of neurotransmitters and neuropeptides [7]. Although many of these have been shown to interact with known natural ligands, several bind ligands that have not been thus far isolated [7]. Structural genomics can also be applied for new drug search. For example, the use of comparative and structural genomics for the search and characterization of new *Mycobacterium tuberculosis* genes, whose products may prove to be important antigens for the development of vaccines or target proteins for remedies against tuberculosis, is considered [8]. In past, long discovery and development times were needed to bring new drugs to market and the bottlenecks at the stages of identifying good lead compounds and optimizing these leads into drug candidates [9]. Structural genomics will hopefully provide opportunities to overcome these bottlenecks and populate the antimicrobial pipeline [9].

C. Chemoinformatics and Drug Search

Sequencing of the human genome along with developments in combinatorial synthesis and high-throughput biological screening provide unparallel opportunities to drug discovery [10]. It has been noted that the increased number of synthesized and annotated compounds did not yield the expected increase in number of viable drug candidates [10]. There are several applications of new computational technologies in chemoinformatics to help drug searching. For example, the identification of three-dimensional pharmacophores from large, heterogeneous data sets is still an unsolved problem [11]. Fortunately, Chen et al developed a novel program, SCAMPI (statistical classification of activities of molecules for pharmacophore identification), for this purpose by combining a fast conformation search with recursive partitioning, a data-mining technique, which can easily handle large data sets [11]. Oloff et al developed a novel structure-based chemoinformatics approach to search for Complimentary Ligands Based on Receptor Information (CoLiBRI) [12]. CoLiBRI is based on the representation of both receptor binding sites and their respective ligands in a space of universal chemical descriptors [12]. The binding site atoms involved in the interaction with ligands are identified by the means of a computational geometry technique known as Delaunay tessellation as applied to X-ray characterized ligand-receptor complexes [12].

BIOINFORMATICS FOR ANTIMALARIAL DRUG SEARCH

1. Bioinformatics Research for Antimalarial Drug Search

1.1 Genomics Research for Antimalarial Drug Search

Quantitative trait loci (QTL) mapping is an effective tool for tracking multi-gene traits by partitioning genetic effects that influence these traits into specific genomic regions [13]. The specific allele forms and their combinations contributed by each parent are, in effect, genetic signatures of their unique evolutionary histories [13]. When alleles conferring drug resistance spread through a population of malaria parasites, they leave characteristic markers in the parasite genome [14]. In addition to resistance genes, per se, a drug resistant parasite carries co-evolved gene combinations comprising a genetic background of drug resistance [13]. Quinine remains effective against *Plasmodium falciparum*, but its decreasing efficacy is documented from different continents. Multiple genes are likely to contribute to the evolution of quinine resistance [15]. Chloroquine-resistant strains of *Plasmodium falciparum* counter the drug by expelling it rapidly via an unknown mechanism [16]. Inheritance data from 16 independent recombinant progeny show that the rapid efflux, chloroquine-resistant phenotype is governed by a single locus within an approximately 400-kilobase region of chromosome [16]. In the absence of explicit biochemical knowledge of this efflux mechanism, reverse genetics provides a powerful approach to the molecular basis of chloroquine resistance [16]. QTL mapping, by superimposing real biological phenotypes on genome sequence, structural polymorphisms, and gene expression data, can provide an alternative, unbiased view of the network of gene actions that build a complex phenotype [13]. To locate genes contributing to QN response variation, Ferdig et al searched a *Plasmodium falciparum* genetic cross for QTL [15]. The mapped segments of Chrs 7 and 5 contain pfcrt, the determinant of chloroquine resistance, and pfmdr1, a gene known to affect QN responses [15]. Association of pfcrt with a QTL of chloroquine resistance supports anecdotal evidence for an evolutionary relationship between chloroquine resistance and reduced quinine sensitivity [15]. The reconstruction of the evolutionary and molecular events underlying chloroquine resistance is important at many levels, including: (i) its potential to assist in the development of rational approaches to thwart future drug resistances; (ii) the stimulation of the use of chloroquine -like compounds in drug combinations for new therapeutic approaches; and (iii) the consideration of how the chloroquine -selected genome will function as the context in which current and future drugs will act, particularly in light of the many reports of multidrug resistance [17]. Through an integrated approach, studies can move beyond the search for markers of resistance to instead characterize the predisposition of parasites to develop new resistances and cross-resistances [13].

Functional genomics can be applied for antimalarial drug search. Combinatorial use of data analysis tools enables powerful data mining queries, such as combining gene and protein expression data to monitor changes through various life-cycle stages [18]. Functional predictions can be used to explore potential targets for antimalarial drug development [18]. The complete annotated genomes of the human parasite *Plasmodium falciparum* and the rodent model *Plasmodium yoelii* is now available thus providing a prediction of their possible gene products [18]. This makes feasible the application of functional genomics to malaria research with the final goal of providing a complete survey of Plasmodium life cycle [19]. Genome-wide approaches to the study of transcriptome or proteome were successfully applied to malaria parasite with the promise for new drug and vaccine candidates in the next future [19]. Another interesting application of functional genomics is for functional study of mitochrondrion of Plasmodium spp. One of the functional roles of the mitochondrion in the parasite is the coordination of pyrimidine biosynthesis, the electron transport system and oxygen utilization via dihydroorotate dehydrogenase and coenzyme Q [20]. Complete sets of genes encoding enzymes of the tricarboxylic acid cycle and the ATP synthase complex are predicted from *Plasmodium falciparum* genomics information [20]. Other metabolic roles of this organelle include membrane potential maintenance, heme and coenzyme Q biosynthesis, and oxidative phosphorylation [20]. Furthermore, the mitochondrion may be a chemotherapeutic target for antimalarial drug development. The antimalarial drug atovaquone targets the mitochondrion [20].

Structural genomics can also be applied for antimalarial drug search. The crystal structure of Pfal009167AAA, a putative ribulose 5-phosphate 3-epimerase (PfalRPE) from *Plasmodium falciparum*, has been determined to 2 A resolution [21]. RPE represents an exciting potential drug target for developing antimalarials because it is involved in the shikimate and the pentose phosphate pathways [21]. This structure is already solved in the framework of the Structural Genomics of Pathogenic Protozoa (SGPP) consortium [21]. Although the conformation of the bound analogue resembles those of ligands bound in the active sites of OMPDC and KGPDC, the identities of the active site residues that coordinate the essential Zn(2+) and participate as acid/base catalysts are not conserved [22]. Akana et al concluded that only the phosphate binding motif located at the ends of the seventh and eighth beta-strands of the (beta/alpha)(8)-barrel is functionally conserved among RPE, OMPDC, and KGPDC, consistent with the hypothesis that the members of the "ribulose phosphate binding" (beta/alpha)(8)-barrel "superfamily" as defined by SCOP have not evolved by evolutionary processes involving the intact (beta/alpha)(8)-barrel [22]. Akana et al proposed that this "superfamily" might result from assembly from smaller modules, including the conserved phosphate binding motif associated with the C-terminal (beta/alpha)(2)-quarter barrel [22].

1.2 Proteomics Research for Antimalarial Drug Search

The search for novel antimalarial drug targets is urgent due to the growing resistance of Plasmodium falciparum parasites to available drugs [23]. The ability to measure accurately comparative levels of protein expression after drug challenge, metabolic stress, developmental programming or other perturbation represents one of the most important goals in post-genomics malaria research [24]. Applied to Plasmodium, proteomics combines high-resolution protein or peptide separation with mass spectrometry and computer software to rapidly identify large numbers of proteins expressed from various stages of parasite development [25]. Proteomic methods can be applied to study sub-cellular localization, cell function, organelle composition, changes in protein expression patterns in response to drug exposure, drug-protein binding and validation of data from genomic annotation and transcript expression studies [25]. Proteases are attractive antimalarial targets because of their indispensable roles in parasite infection and development, especially in the processes of host erythrocyte rupture/invasion and hemoglobin degradation [23]. Wu et al represents an initial effort to identify a set of expressed, active, and essential proteases as targets for inhibitor-based drug design based on proteomics techniques [23]. Recently, Nirmalan et al described a simple and robust quantitative methodology that was ideally suited to in vitro experiments designed to study changes in the proteome of the most important of the human parasites, the lethal species *Plasmodium falciparum* [24]. According to this work, the metabolic labeling technique uses parasite uptake of heavy isotope-containing isoleucine during normal growth followed by two-dimensional separation of individual proteins and mass spectrometry [24]. Recent high-throughput proteomic approaches have provided a wealth of protein expression data on *Plasmodium falciparum*, while smaller-scale studies examining specific drug-related hypotheses are also appearing [25].

2. Chemoinformatics Research Antimalarial drug Search

New antimalarial targets are required to allow the discovery of chemically diverse, effective drugs. The search for such new targets and new drug chemotypes will likely be helped by the advent of functional genomics and structure-based drug design [26]. After validation of the putative targets as those capable of providing effective and safe drugs, targets can be used as the basis for screening compounds in order to identify new leads, which, in turn, will qualify for lead optimization work [26]. The combined use of combinatorial chemistry to generate large numbers of structurally diverse compounds and of high throughput screening systems to speed up the testing of compounds will help to optimize the process [26]. For example, the 4-aminoquinolines have provided a number of useful antimalarials, and *Plasmodium falciparum*, the causative organism for the most deadly form of human malaria, is generally slow to develop resistance to these drugs [27]. Therefore, diverse screening libraries of quinolines continue to be useful for antimalarial drug discovery [27]. The effects of these substitutions were evaluated by screening this library for activity against *Plasmodium falciparum*, revealing four potent compounds active against drug-resistant strains [27].

A consideration on molecular mechanics of antimalarial drug is also useful for further development of new antimalarial drug. The selection of antimalarial drugs depends on the species and the reported resistance pattern in each setting. The mechanism of action of artemisinin compounds consists of two important steps: (a) activation and (b) alkylation. In the activation step by iron, there are two possible pathways for developing C-4 free radical: (a) 1.5 H-shift and (b) C-C cleavage. Recently, Wiwanitkit performed a quantum chemical analysis of the activation reaction of artemisinin by the two alternative pathways [28]. According to this study, the required energy for compound formation in C-C cleavage is more than that for C-O cleavage [28]. It can be noted that the C-C cleavage pathway is less preferable, implying that the 1.5 H-shift should be the more common phenomenon [28].

However, compounds that can easily proceed along the pathway 1 have high activity [29]. Therefore, both pathways are important for antimalarial activity. Moreover, effective discrimination between high and low activity compounds using EA1, deltaE1, and deltaE(1A-2A) was accomplished [29].

Finally, reconstructing synthetic metabolic pathways in microbes holds great promise for the production of pharmaceuticals in large-scale fermentations [30]. By recreating biosynthetic pathways in bacteria, complex molecules traditionally harvested from scarce natural resources can be produced in microbial cultures [30]. Recently, Newman et al reported on a strain of Escherichia coli containing a heterologous, nine-gene biosynthetic pathway for the production of the terpene amorpha-4,11-diene, a precursor to the anti-malarial drug artemisinin [30].

References

[1] Ivanov AS, Veselovsky AV, Dubanov AV, Skvortsov VS. Bioinformatics platform development: from gene to lead compound. *Methods Mol Biol.* 2006;316:389-431.
[2] Chang PL. Clinical bioinformatics. *Chang Gung Med J.* 2005;28:201-11.
[3] Attwood PK. The quest to deduce protein function from sequence: the role of pattern databases. *Int J Biochem Cell Biol.* 2000;32:139-55.
[4] Pany YP. In silico drug discovery: solving the "target-rich and lead-poor" imbalance using the genome-to-drug-lead paradigm. *Clin Pharmacol Ther.* 2007;81:30-4.
[5] Bansal AK. Bioinformatics in microbial biotechnology--a mini review. *Microb Cell Fact.* 2005;4:19.
[6] Wiwanitkit V. Analysis of Mycobacterium leprae genome: in silico searching for drug targets. *Southeast Asian J Trop Med Public Health.* 2005;36 Suppl 4:225-7.
[7] Civelli O, Nothacker HP. Functional genomics and the discovery of new drug targets. *Diabetes Technol Ther.* 1999;1:71-6.
[8] Kariagina AS, Naroditskii BS, Apt AS, Gintsburg AL. Genomics and gene engineering: rationale to the development of new means of tuberculosis control. *Zh Mikrobiol Epidemiol Immunobiol.* 2004;(4):94-101.
[9] Schmid MB. Seeing is believing: the impact of structural genomics on antimicrobial drug discovery. *Nat Rev Microbiol.* 2004;2:739-46.
[10] Balakin KV, Kozintsev AV, Kiselyov AS, Savchuk NP.Rational design approaches to chemical libraries for hit identification. *Curr Drug Discov Technol.* 2006;3:49-65.
[11] Chen X, Rusinko A 3rd, Tropsha A, Young SS. Automated pharmacophore identification for large chemical data sets. *J Chem Inf Comput Sci.* 1999;39:887-96.
[12] Oloff S, Zhang S, Sukumar N, Breneman C, Tropsha A. Chemometric analysis of ligand receptor complementarity: identifying Complementary Ligands Based on Receptor Information (CoLiBRI). *J Chem Inf Model.* 2006;46:844-51.
[13] Sen S, Ferdig M. QTL analysis for discovery of genes involved in drug responses. *Curr Drug Targets Infect Disord.* 2004;4:53-63.
[14] Anderson TJ. Mapping drug resistance genes in Plasmodium falciparum by genome-wide association. *Curr Drug Targets Infect Disord.* 2004;4:65-78.

[15] Ferdig MT, Cooper RA, Mu J, Deng B, Joy DA, Su XZ, Wellems TE. Dissecting the loci of low-level quinine resistance in malaria parasites. *Mol Microbiol.* 2004;52:985-97.

[16] Wellems TE, Walker-Jonah A, Panton LJ. Genetic mapping of the chloroquine-resistance locus on Plasmodium falciparum chromosome 7. *Proc Natl Acad Sci U S A.* 1991;88:3382-6.

[17] Cooper RA, Hartwig CL, Ferdig MT. pfcrt is more than the Plasmodium falciparum chloroquine resistance gene: a functional and evolutionary perspective. *Acta Trop.* 2005;94:170-80.

[18] Di Girolamo F, Raggi C, Bultrini E, Lanfrancotti A, Silvestrini F, Sargiacomo M, Birago C, Pizzi E, Alano P, Ponzi M. Functional genomics, new tools in malaria research. *Ann Ist Super Sanita.* 2005;41:469-77.

[19] Fraunholz MJ, Roos DS. PlasmoDB: exploring genomics and post-genomics data of the malaria parasite, Plasmodium falciparum. *Redox Rep.* 2003;8:317-20.

[20] Krungkrai J. The multiple roles of the mitochondrion of the malarial parasite. *Parasitology.* 2004;129:511-24.

[21] Caruthers J, Bosch J, Buckner F, Van Voorhis W, Myler P, Worthey E, Mehlin C, Boni E, DeTitta G, Luft J, Lauricella A, Kalyuzhniy O, Anderson L, Zucker F, Soltis M, Hol WG.Structure of a ribulose 5-phosphate 3-epimerase from Plasmodium falciparum. *Proteins.* 2006;62:338-42.

[22] Akana J, Fedorov AA, Fedorov E, Novak WR, Babbitt PC, Almo SC, Gerlt JA. D-Ribulose 5-phosphate 3-epimerase: functional and structural relationships to members of the ribulose-phosphate binding (beta/alpha)8-barrel superfamily. *Biochemistry.* 2006;45:2493-503.

[23] Wu Y, Wang X, Liu X, Wang Y. Data-mining approaches reveal hidden families of proteases in the genome of malaria parasite. *Genome Res.* 2003;13:601-16.

[24] Nirmalan N, Sims PF, Hyde JE. Quantitative proteomics of the human malaria parasite Plasmodium falciparum and its application to studies of development and inhibition. *Mol Microbiol.* 2004;52:1187-99.

[25] Cooper RA, Carucci DJ. Proteomic approaches to studying drug targets and resistance in Plasmodium. *Curr Drug Targets Infect Disord.* 2004;4:41-51.

[26] Olliaro PL, Yuthavong Y. An overview of chemotherapeutic targets for antimalarial drug discovery. *Pharmacol Ther.* 1999;81:91-110.

[27] Madrid PB, Wilson NT, DeRisi JL, Guy RK. Parallel synthesis and antimalarial screening of a 4-aminoquinoline library. *J Comb Chem.* 2004;6:437-42.

[28] Wiwanitkit V. Quantum chemical analysis of alternative pathways for iron activation step for artemisinin, a new antimalarial drug. *J Infect.* 2006;53:148-51.

[29] Tonmunphean S, Parasuk V, Kokpol S. Effective discrimination of antimalarial potency of artemisinin compounds based on quantum chemical calculations of their reaction mechanism. *Bioorg Med Chem.* 2006;14:2082-8.

[30] Newman JD, Marshall J, Chang M, Nowroozi F, Paradise E, Pitera D, Newman KL, Keasling JD.High-level production of amorpha-4,11-diene in a two-phase partitioning bioreactor of metabolically engineered Escherichia coli. *Biotechnol Bioeng.* 2006;95:684-91.

Chapter 14

MALARIA IN ANDAMAN ISLANDS

ABSTRACT

Andaman Islands is an island area of Southeast Asia. It is an area lining in Andaman Sea. In this area, there are numerous sea tribers. Also, it is considered as an area with high public health and social problems. In this article, the situation and items relating to malaria in Andaman Islands will be discussed.

INTRODUCTION TO ANDAMAN ISLANDS

Andaman Islands is an island area of Southeast Asia. It is an area lining in Andaman Sea. It is a famous area containing several sea resorts. In this area, there are numerous sea tribers. The recent Southeast Asian Tsunami directly hit to the seashore of Andaman sea and cause several damages. Indonesia's devastating Sumatra-Andaman earthquake on 26 December 2004 was 2.5 times larger than initial reports suggested--second only to the 1960 Chilean earthquake in recorded magnitude [1]. The first event generated a tsunami that caused more than 283,000 deaths. Fault slip of up to 15 meters occurred near Banda Aceh, Sumatra, but to the north, along the Nicobar and Andaman Islands, rapid slip was much smaller [2]. Andaman Islands is considered as an area with high public health and social problems. Several infectious diseases, drug addiction as well as poverty are common in this area. In this article, the situation and items relating to malaria in Andaman Islands will be discussed.

IMPORTANT PROBLEMS OF MALARIA IN ANDAMAN ISLANDS

A. Malaria and Sea

Climatic factors influence the emergence and reemergence of infectious diseases, in addition to multiple human, biological, and ecological determinants[3]. Island is a type of geography which a limitation of land area due to the sea.The impact of islands on the population structure of *Anopheles flavirostris*(Ludlow) (Diptera: Culicidae), the primary malaria vector in the Philippines, wasAssessed by Foley et al [4]. According to this work [4], sea barriers appeared to be important for *An. flavirostris* population structure. Our results suggest that endemic island malaria vector species need to be considered before any generalizations are made about the population structure of primary and secondary vectors [4]. Air, sea and land transport networks continue to expand in reach, speed of travel and volume of passengers and goods carried [5]. Pathogens and their vectors can now move further, faster and in greater numbers than ever before [5]. Tatem et al proposed that *An. gambiae* had rarely spread from Africa, which might partly due to the low volume of sea traffic from the continent and, until very recently, a European destination for most flights [5].

At present, scuba diving vacations in tropical surroundings belong to the repertoire of most divers [6]. In addition to carefully making travel plans and taking care of the necessary vaccinations and appropriate malaria prophylaxis, the following points also must be observed [6]. Since many sea resorts are in the forest area, the concern of getting malaria from mosquito bite should be set by all travelers [6 – 7]. Transverse furrows, or Beau's lines, noted in the fingernails is an important manifestation in numerous medical conditions such as typhus, rheumatic fever, malaria, myocardial infarction, and other severe metabolic stresses [8]. Of interest, this can also be seen in the patients following a deep saturation dive [8].

B. Malaria and Sea Tribers

Sea triber is an original population group within Southeast Asia [9]. The dispersal of southern Chinese into mainland Southeast Asia may have included a westward expansion and colonization of the islands of the Andaman Sea [10]. Andaman and Nicobar Islands, union territory of India are inhabited by more than aboriginal tribes [11]. Malaria is one of important infectious diseases in Andaman Islands [12]. Studies on bioecology of An. philippinensis a vector of malaria was carried out in eight islands of the Andaman group [13]. The breeding association of *An. philippinensis* was found with other seven anopheline species in different breeding habitats [13]. According to the study of Das et al, there was absence of malarial parasite *Plasmodium vivax* infection though *Plasmodium falciparum* infection was present in 27.59% of cases [11]. A very high frequency of Fy (a-b-) in the Jarawa tribe from all the four jungle areas of Andaman Islands along with total absence of *P. vivax* infections suggests the selective advantage offered to Fy (a-b-) individuals against *P vivax* infection [11]. In addition, the antifolate drug pressure is very high in the island, which should be a cause of concern for the malaria control program in this area [14].

C. Malaria and Tsunami

There are some interesting reports on malaria after tsunami attacked to Andaman Islands. Because of great intervening distances, international medical relief activities in catastrophic, sudden-onset disasters often do not begin until days 5-7 after the precipitating event. There is a risk of vector abundance with enhanced malaria transmission potential, due to the vastness of these tsunami-created breeding grounds and likelihood of them becoming permanent due to continued flooding in view of land subsidence [15]. The close proximity of the houses and paucity of cattle may lead to a higher degree of man/vector contact causing a threat of malaria outbreak in this densely populated area [15]. Measures to prevent the possible outbreak of malaria in this tsunami-affected area should be discussed [15]. According to the record public health problems exist in the community in the week after the tsunami disaster in Papua New Guinea, no outbreak of communicable disease occurred, despite the presence of risk factors such as the dense concentration of affected people and the constant prevalence of malaria and diarrhea [16]. Similar to the recent Southeast Asian tsunami, the record from Sri Lanka showed that the environmental changes caused by the tsunami are unlikely to enhance breeding of the principal vector, and, given the present low parasite reservoir, the likelihood of a malaria outbreak is low [17]. There were no indications of increased malaria vector abundance [18]. Overall it is concluded that the tsunami has not negatively influenced the malaria situation in Sri Lanka [18].

Epidemiology of Malaria in Andaman Islands Area

1. Andaman Seashores of Thailand

Indeed, malaria is well controlled in the Andaman seashores ofThailand. However, the emerging of malaria due to the migration from Myanmar is noted. It should be noted that the efficacy of mefloquine alone in Ranong has significantly dropped for a few years [19 - 20]. There is an interesting on population genetic structure of *Anopheles maculatus* in Thailand [21]. According to this study, gene flow is restricted between proximal collections located on different sides of the Phuket mountain range [21].

2. Andaman Seashore of Myanmar

It is expected that the prevalence of malaria among Andaman seashore in the Southern part of Myanmar is very high. However, there are only a few reports on this topic. The bionomics of vectors in this area is similar to that of Andaman seashore of Thailand [22].

3. Andaman Islands of India

As previously mentioned, malaria is still important problem for Andaman islands of India. Based on dihydrofolate reductase - dihydropteroate synthetase mutations, the expected level of sulfadoxine and pyrimethamine resistance was highest in India in Car Nicobar in the Andaman islands of India [23].

References

[1] Stein S, Okal EA. Seismology: speed and size of the Sumatra earthquake. *Nature*. 2005;434:581-2.

[2] Lay T, Kanamori H, Ammon CJ, Nettles M, Ward SN, Aster RC, Beck SL, Bilek SL, Brudzinski MR, Butler R, DeShon HR, Ekstrom G, Satake K, Sipkin S. The great Sumatra-Andaman earthquake of 26 December 2004. *Science*. 2005;308:1127-33.

[3] Patz JA, Epstein PR, Burke TA, Balbus JM. Global climate change and emerging infectious diseases. *JAMA*. 1996;275:217-23.

[4] Foley DH, Torres EP. Population structure of an island malaria vector. *Med Vet Entomol*. 2006;20:393-401.

[5] Tatem AJ, Rogers DJ, Hay SI. Global transport networks and infectious disease spread. *Adv Parasitol*. 2006;62:293-343.

[6] Muth CM, Muller P, Kemmer A. Medical aspects of diving in the tropics. *MMW Fortschr Med*. 2005;147:28-32.

[7] Robinet C. Scuba diving in the tropics. *Med Trop* (Mars). 1999;59:225-6.

[8] Toovey S. Malaria chemoprophylaxis advice: survey of South African community pharmacists' knowledge and practices. *J Travel Med*. 2006;13:161-5.

[9] Endicott P, Gilbert MT, Stringer C, Lalueza-Fox C, Willerslev E, Hansen AJ, Cooper A. The genetic origins of the Andaman Islanders. *Am J Hum Genet*. 2003;72:178-84.

[10] Prasad BV, Ricker CE, Watkins WS, Dixon ME, Rao BB, Naidu JM, Jorde LB, Bamshad M. Mitochondrial DNA variation in Nicobarese Islanders. : *Hum Biol*. 2001;73:715-25.

[11] Das MK, Singh SS, Adak T, Vasantha K, Mohanty D. The Duffy blood groups of Jarawas - the primitive and vanishing tribe of Andaman and Nicobar Islands of India. *Transfus Med*. 2005;15:237-40.

[12] Basu SK. A health profile of tribal India. *Health Millions*. 1994;2:12-4.

[13] Das MK, Nagpal BN, Srivastava A, Ansari MA. Bioecology of An. philippinensis in Andaman group of islands. *J Vector Borne Dis*. 2003;40:43-8.

[14] Ahmed A, Das MK, Dev V, Saifi MA, Wajihullah, Sharma YD. Quadruple mutations in dihydrofolate reductase of Plasmodium falciparum isolates from Car Nicobar Island, India. *Antimicrob Agents Chemother*. 2006;50:1546-9.

[15] Krishnamoorthy K, Jambulingam P, Natarajan R, Shriram AN, Das PK, Sehgal S. Altered environment and risk of malaria outbreak in South Andaman, Andaman & Nicobar Islands, India affected by tsunami disaster. *Malar J*. 2005;4:30.

[16] Asari Y, Koido Y, Nakamura K, Yamamoto Y, Ohta M. Analysis of medical needs on day 7 after the tsunami disaster in Papua New Guinea. *Prehospital Disaster Med*. 2000;15:9-13.

[17] Briet OJ, Galappaththy GN, Konradsen F, Amerasinghe PH, Amerasinghe FP. Maps of the Sri Lanka malaria situation preceding the tsunami and key aspects to be considered in the emergency phase and beyond. *Malar J*. 2005;4:8.

[18] Briet OJ, Galappaththy GN, Amerasinghe PH, Konradsen F. Malaria in Sri Lanka: one year post-tsunami. *Malar J*. 2006;5:42.

[19] Rojanawatsirivet C, Congpuong K, Vijaykadga S, Thongphua S, Thongsri K, Bangchang KN, Wilairatana P, Wernsdorfer WH. Declining mefloquine sensitivity of Plasmodium falciparum along the Thai-Myanmar border. *Southeast Asian J Trop Med Public Health*. 2004;35:560-5.

[20] Rojanawatsirivej C, Vijaykadga S, Amklad I, Wilairatna P, Looareesuwan S. Monitoring the therapeutic efficacy of antimalarials against uncomplicated falciparum malaria in Thailand. *Southeast Asian J Trop Med Public Health*. 2003;34:536-41.

[21] Rongnopaurt P, Rodpradit P, Kongsawadworakul P, Sithiprasasna R, Linthicum KJ. Population genetic structure of Anopheles maculatus in Thailand. *J Am Mosq Control Assoc*. 2006;22:192-7.

[22] Ool TT, Storch V, Becker N. Review of the anopheline mosquitoes of Myanmar. *J Vector Ecol.* 2004;29:21-40.

[23] Ahmed A, Lumb V, Das MK, Dev V, Wajihullah, Sharma YD. Prevalence of mutations associated with higher levels of sulfadoxine-pyrimethamine resistance in Plasmodium falciparum isolates from Car Nicobar Island and Assam, India. *Antimicrob Agents Chemother.* 2006; 50:3934-8.

Chapter 15

Malaria and Other Common Infectious Diseases

Abstract

In addition to malaria, there are other important tropical infectious diseases. In this article, the author summarizes the correlation between malaria and other common infectious diseases. Syphilis, tuberculosis as well as human immunodeficiency virus infection are focused.

Malaria and Syphilis

Syphilis is a well-known sexually transmitted disease found around the world. Malaria and syphilis are endemic in many regions of the world, and co-infection with the two pathogens is common [1]. The interaction between both infections within an co-infection episode is an interesting topic in infectious medicine and becomes a new interesting research topic. N'Gom et al found that HIV-2 infection is co-infected with syphilis is associated with a further lowering of CD4+ count, suggesting a worse suppression of the immune system while co-infection with malaria is associated with a modest immune disturbance [2]. Indeed, syphilis poses the nature of immune suppression that leads chronicity Similar, immune suppression by malaria is also noted [4]. Long-term immunity to malaria infection may be affected by an IFN-gamma-mediated depletion of parasite-specific CD4+ T cells during infection [5]. During the co-infection, the synergistic effect between each other can be expected. However, a study on the proteins' expression in an episode of co-infection is warranted. To study the interaction between both infections, the new development in bioinformatics can be applied. Here, the author used a new gene ontology technology to predict the pathway of CD4+ suppression in an episode of co-infection. The author used PubMed (ww.pubmed.com) search to find the document proposing the pathway for CD4+ suppression in both malaria and syphilis. Then the interactions among the pathways are searched. The final resulted interaction map is then created. Derived mechanisms for CD4+ suppression in malaria and syphilis are presented in Table 1. The final resulted interaction map is presented in Figure 1.

Table 1. Derived Mechanism for CD4+ Suppression in Malaria and Syphilis.

Diseases	Mechanisms
Malaria	Modulating dendritic cell function by hemozoin [6]
	Inhibit interleukin-2 (IL-2) secreted by CD4+ [7]
	Nitric oxide production [8 - 9]
Syphilis	Inhibit interleukin-2 (IL-2) secreted by CD4+ [10 - 11]
	Impairment of mitogenic factor [12 - 13]
	Nitric oxide production [14]

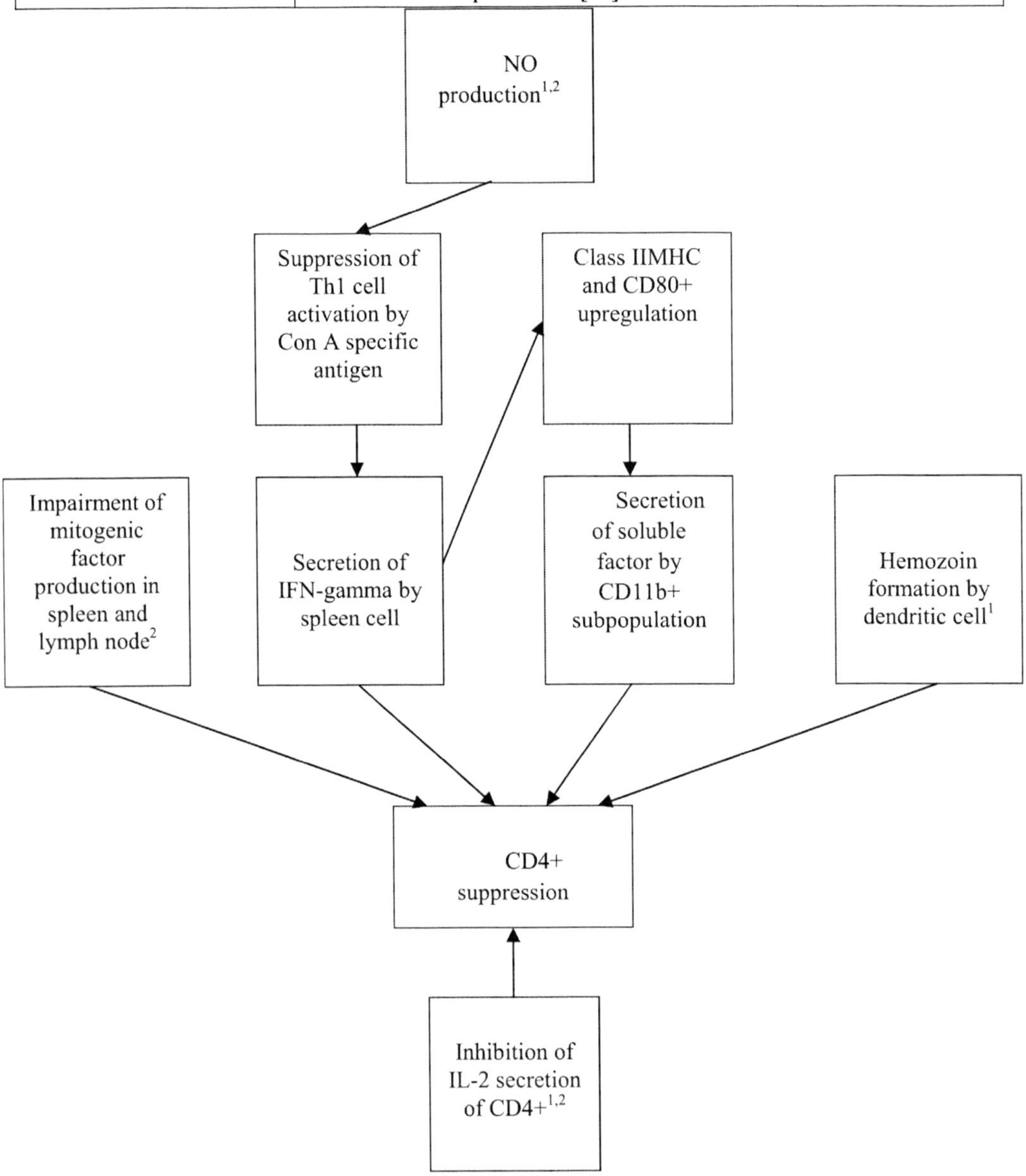

(1 = mechanism in malaria, 2 = mechanism in syphilis)

Figure 1. Pathway for CD4+ suppression due to syphilis and malaria co-infection.

New developments have forced a re-evaluation of our understanding on tropical infections. Both malaria and syphilis are important tropical infectious diseases. The co-occurrence between these two diseases can be expected. A large proportion of people with latent syphilis live in malaria-endemic areas, so co-infection with these two organisms is likely to be common. Aberration in pathogenesis of infection in an episode of malaria and syphilis co-occurrence is interesting and becomes a new focus in tropical medicine. The aberration in immunological process is believed to be important part in the pathogenesis of co-infection. Here, the author studied the pathogenesis of CD4+ suppression in malaria-syphilis co-infection. The pathway ontology technique is used. This technique is a new concept and used in some recent molecular biological studies. Of interest, the author found that there are some immune suppression process that can be found both in syphilis and malaria. The mentioned processes are inhibit interleukin-2 (IL-2) secreted by CD4+ [7, 10 - 11] and nitric oxide production [8 – 9, 14]. In the co-infection, the synergy to increase the immune suppression can be expected. However, further experimental studies are needed before making a conclusion on this topic. The finding in this study is not only supports the previous knowledge on malaria and syphilis but also gives the new view on the pathogenesis of co-infection.

MALARIA AND TUBERCULOSIS

Malaria and tuberculosis are endemic in many regions of the world, and coinfection with the two pathogens is common. The interaction between both infections within an coinfection episode is an interesting topic in infectious medicine and becomes a new interesting research topic. Page et al said that tuberculosis-induced potentiation of type 1 immune responses is associated with protection against lethal murine malaria [15]. The protective process is believed to relate to gamma interferon induction [15]. This induction of cellular immune responses is related to ATP-binding protein (ATPBP) of Plasmodium species [16]. Zheng et al found that heat shock protein 70 (HSP70) from *Mycobacterium tuberculosis* was associated with the induction of a strong humoral and cellular response directed against *Plasmodium falciparum* [17]. During the coinfection, the protective effect between each other was noted and has been studied for a few years [15 – 17]. However, a study on the proteins' expression in an episode of coinfection is warranted. To study the interaction between both infections, the new development in bioinformatics can be applied.

Here, the author used a new gene ontology technology to predict the molecular function of HSP70 and ATPBP in an episode of coinfection. The database PubMed was used for data mining of the amino acid sequence for HSP70 and ATPBP. The author performs prediction of molecular function and biological process of HSP70 and ATPBP using a novel gene ontology prediction tool, GoFigure [18]. GoFigure is an computational algorithm tool which is recently developed in gene ontology [18]. The prediction of molecular function were presented and compared. From searching of the database, sequence of *M.* HSP70 and ATPBP can be derived and used for further study. Using GoFigure server, the molecular function in HSP70 and ATPBP is predicted. Of interest, HSP70 and ATPBP share a common molecular function as ATP binding resulting from purine nucleotide binding. Therefore, a competitive antagonist effect between both molecules can be expected. This finding can be a good explanation for the protective effect between each other in malaria-tuberculosis co-infection. Indeed, the structural homology between both studied molecules was reported in a recent study by Garsia et al [19]. However, further experimental studies are needed before making a conclusion on this topic. The finding in this study is not only supports the previous knowledge on malaria and tuberculosis but also gives the new view on the pathogenesis of co-infection.

MALARIA AND HUMAN IMMUNODEFICIENCY VIRUS INFECTION

HIV seropositive people staying in malaria endemic areas are at risk of developing severe malaria [20]. Malaria prevention using insecticide-treated bednets and indoor residual house spraying may be the best available options for these people [20]. Some medical practice for malaria, especially for blood transfusion in treatment of children with anemia from malaria can be the route of HIV infection, especially in Africa [21 - 22]. On the other hand, some risk behaviors for HIV infection increase the risk of malaria. Bastos *et al* noted that new outbreaks of cases of HIV and malaria were likely to occur among Brazilian injecting drug users (IDUs), and might conceivably contribute to the development of treatment-resistant strains of malaria in this population [22]. They proposed that health professionals should be alert to this possibility, which could also eventually occur in IDU networks in developed countries [23]. Co-infection might also have facilitated the geographic expansion of malaria in areas where HIV prevalence is high [24]. Abu-Raddad proposed that transient and repeated increases in HIV viral load resulting from recurrent co-infection with malaria might be an important factor in promoting the spread of HIV in sub-Saharan Africa [24]. The coexistence of malaria and HIV infection beyond inhabitants of sub-Saharan Africa, South America and South-East Asia arises a question whether there is an interaction between these two infections that bring the change of the pathogenesis [25].

Diagnosis of co-infection is usually by detection of malaria parasites in red blood cells and detection of positive HIV serology. There is no reported on the effect of co-infection on the diagnostic test. Slutsker and Marston mentioned that malaria wais associated with increases in HIV viral load that, while modest, might impact HIV progression or the risk of HIV transmission [26]. HIV-infected persons are at increased risk for clinical malaria; the risk is greatest when immune suppression is advanced [26]. In tropical countries, immunosupression due to HIV infection has resulted in changes in the clinical presentation of endemic infections [27]. Adults with advanced HIV may be at risk for failure of malaria treatment, especially with sulfa-based therapies [26]. According to the study of Van Geertruyden et al, HIV-1-infected patients with malaria with a CD4 cell count <300 cells/microL have a higher risk of experiencing a recrudescent infection, compared with those with a CD4 cell count >or=300 cells/microL or without HIV-1 infection [28]. Slutsker and Marston mentioned that people with HIV should use cotrimoxazole and insecticide treated mosquito nets [26]. Malaria prevention is particularly important for pregnant women with HIV, although more information is needed about the best combination of strategies for prevention [26]. Increased numbers of doses of intermittent preventive treatment during pregnancy can reduce the risk of placental malaria in women with HIV [26]. Sulfadoxine-pyrimethamine should be prescribed cautiously in women concurrently receiving daily neviripine and/or zidovudine, and should be avoided in women on daily co-trimoxazole [29]. This should also be applied for the HIV-infected traveler [30].

REFERENCES

[1] Harris VK, Nair SC, Das PK, Sitaram U, Bose YN, Sudarsanam A, Mathai E. Prevalence of syphilis and parasitic infection among blood donors in a tertiary-care centre in southern India. *Ann Trop Med Parasitol.* 1999;93:763-5.

[2] N'Gom PT, Jaffar S, Ricard D, Wilkins A, Ariyoshi K, Morgan G, Da Silva AP, Whittle HC. Immune stimulation by syphilis and malaria in HIV-2-infected and uninfected villagers in West Africa. Br *J Biomed Sci.* 1997;54:251-5.

[3] Wright DJ, Grimble AS. Why is the infectious stage of syphilis prolonged? *Br J Vener Dis.* 1974;50:45-9.

[4] Hisaeda H, Yasutomo K, Himeno K. Malaria: immune evasion by parasites. *Int J Biochem Cell Biol.* 2005;37:700-6.

[5] Xu H, Wipasa J, Yan H, Zeng M, Makobongo MO, Finkelman FD, Kelso A, Good MF. The mechanism and significance of deletion of parasite-specific CD4(+) T cells in malaria infection. *J Exp Med.* 2002;195:881-92.

[6] Millington OR, Di Lorenzo C, Phillips RS, Garside P, Brewer JM. Suppression of adaptive immunity to heterologous antigens during *Plasmodium* infection through hemozoin-induced failure of dendritic cell function. *J Biol.* 2006;5:5.

[7] Luyendyk J, Olivas OR, Ginger LA, Avery AC. Antigen-presenting cell function during Plasmodium yoelii infection. *Infect Immun.* 2002;70:2941-9.

[8] Taylor-Robinson AW. Inhibition of IL-2 production by nitric oxide: a novel self-regulatory mechanism for Th1 cell proliferation. *Immunol Cell Biol.* 1997;75:167-75.

[9] Nahrevanian H, Gholizadeh J, Farahmand M, Assmar M, Sharifi K, Ayatollahi Mousavi SA, Abolhassani M. Nitric oxide induction as a novel immunoepidemiological target in malaria-infected patients from endemic areas of the Islamic Republic of Iran. *Scand J Clin Lab Invest.* 2006;66:201-9.

[10] Tomai MA, Elmquist BJ, Warmka SM, Fitzgerald TJ. Macrophage-mediated suppression of con A-induced IL-2 production in spleen cells from syphilitic rabbits. *J Immunol.* 1989; 143: 309-14.

[11] Baker-Zander SA, Sell S, Lukehart SA. Serum regulation of in vitro lymphocyte responses in early experimental syphilis. *Infect Immun.* 1982;37: 568-78.

[12] Wicher V, Wicher K. In vitro cell response of Treponema pallidum-infected rabbits. III. Impairment in production of lymphocyte mitogenic factor. *Clin Exp Immunol.* 1977;29:496-500.

[13] Maret SM, Baseman JB, Folds JD. Cell-mediated immunity in Treponema pallidum infected rabbits: in vitro response of splenic and lymph node lymphocytes to mitogens and specific antigens. *Clin Exp Immunol.* 1980;39:38-43.

[14] Lusiak M, Podwinska J. Interleukin 10 and its role in the regulation of the cell-mediated immune response in syphilis. *Arch Immunol Ther Exp* (Warsz). 2001;49:417-21.

[15] Page KR, Jedlicka AE, Fakheri B, Noland GS, Kesavan AK, Scott AL, Kumar N, Manabe YC. Mycobacterium-induced potentiation of type 1 immune responses and protection against malaria are host specific. *Infect Immun.* 2005;73:8369-80.

[16] Riley EM, Williamson KC, Greenwood BM, Kaslow DC. Human immune recognition of recombinant proteins representing discrete domains of the Plasmodium falciparum gamete surface protein, Pfs230. *Parasite Immunol.* 1995;17:11-9.

[17] Zheng C, Xie P, Chen Y. Immune response induced by recombinant BCG expressing merozoite surface antigen 2 from Plasmodium falciparum. *Vaccine.* 2001;20:914-9.

[18] Khan S, Situ G, Decker K, Schmidt CJ. GoFigure: automated Gene Ontology

[19] annotation. *Bioinformatics* 2003;19:2484-5.

[20] Garsia SJ, Hellqvist L, Booth RJ, Radford AJ, Britton WJ, Astbury L, Trent RJ, Basten A. Homology of the 70-kilodalton antigens from Mycobacterium leprae and Mycobacterium bovis with the Mycobacterium tuberculosis 71-kilodalton antigen and with the conserved heat shock protein 70 of eucaryotes. *Infect Immun.* 1989;57:204-12.

[21] Chirenda J, Murugasampillay S. Malaria and HIV co-infection: available evidence, gaps and possible interventions. *Cent Afr J Med.* 2003;49:66-71.

[22] Piot P, Carael M. Epidemiological and sociological aspects of HIV-infection in developing countries. *Br Med Bull.* 1988;44:68-88.

[23] Fleming AF. HIV and blood transfusion in sub-Saharan Africa. *Transfus Sci.* 1997;18:167-79.

[24] Bastos FI, Barcellos C, Lowndes CM, Friedman SR. Co-infection with malaria and HIV in injecting drug users in Brazil: a new challenge to public health? *Addiction.* 1999; 94: 1165-74.

[25] Abu-Raddad LJ, Patnaik P, Kublin JG. Dual infection with HIV and malaria fuels the spread of both diseases in sub-Saharan Africa. *Science.* 2006;314:1603-6.

[26] Siwak E, Kowalczuk-Kot A, Pogorzelska J. Malaria and HIV co-infection. *Wiad Parazytol.* 2006;52:9-11.

[27] Slutsker L, Marston BJ. HIV and malaria: interactions and implications. *Curr Opin Infect Dis.* 2007;20:3-10.

[28] Suri V, Bhalla A, Sharma N, Jain S, Varma S. HIV immunosupression and malaria: is there a correlation? *Indian J Med Sci.* 2006;60:376-9.

[29] McCarthy AE, Mileno MD. Prevention and treatment of travel-related infections in compromised hosts. *Curr Opin Infect Dis.* 2006;19:450-5.

[30] Brentlinger PE, Behrens CB, Micek MA. Challenges in the concurrent management of malaria and HIV in pregnancy in sub-Saharan Africa. *Lancet Infect Dis.* 2006;6:100-11.

[31] Van Geertruyden JP, Mulenga M, Mwananyanda L, Chalwe V, Moerman F, Chilengi R, Kasongo W, Van Overmeir C, Dujardin JC, Colebunders R, Kestens L, D'Alessandro U. HIV-1 immune suppression and antimalarial treatment outcome in Zambian adults with uncomplicated malaria. *J Infect Dis.* 2006;194:917-25.

Chapter 16

REVIEW OF MALARIA RESEARCH IN MALAYSIA

Jamaiah Ibrahim*

*Department of Parasitology, Faculty of Medicine, University Malaya
50603, Kuala Lumpur Malaysia

ABSTRACT

Malaria is a disease that has hampered economic development in the country. In Malaysia, organized anti malaria campaign began in 1901 through integrated parasitological and entomological surveillance systems, followed by the development of permanent anti-larval work. Review of malaria research in Malaysia will be presented in this chapter.

INTRODUCTION

Malaria remains an important public health issue in remote areas of Malaysia. The high morbidity to malaria is because this country is located within the equatorial zone with high temperature and humidity, which is important for the transmission of this disease. It affects mainly the rural and semi-rural population, especially in the areas where clearing of jungles for development is going on. In Peninsular Malaysia, infection rates are highest among the aboriginal Orang Asli minority group and soldiers. Illegal land scheme workers, often foreigners, also exhibit high infection rates. At highest risk are forest workers (loggers, rattan collectors and forest product gatherers), followed by plantation workers and other aboriginal communities [1]. Thomas *et al* [2], Oothuman [3], Mak *et al*, [4], Rahman *et al*, [5] and Ministry of Health Malaysia [6] also reported high rate of infection among the indigenous Orang Asli.

The most common species of malarial parasite in Malaysia is *Plasmodium falciparum* followed closely by *Plasmodium vivax* and few reported cases of *Plasmodium malariae* . There was no reported case of *Plasmodium ovale*. [3-4, 7 – 14].

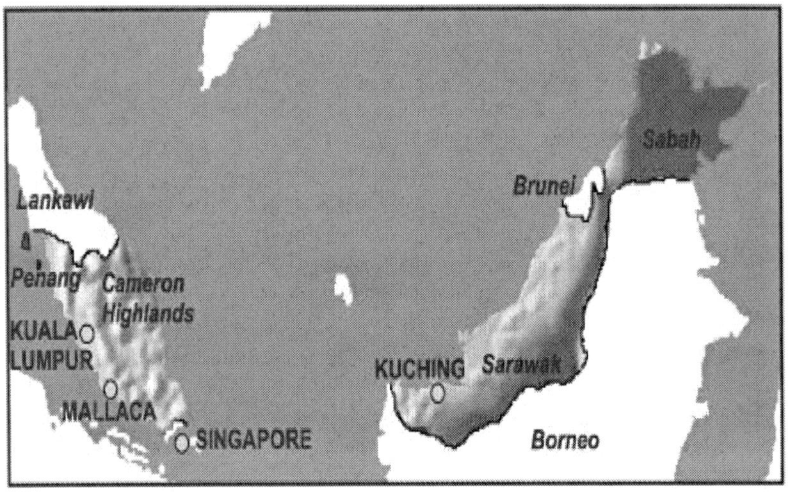

Figure 1: Reported malaria cases in Malaysia in 2005 (Red) (Source internet).

Anopheles maculatus mosquito is the main malaria vector in northern Peninsular Malaysia. In Sarawak, the main malaria vectors are *An. leucosphyrus* and *An. donaldi*, which breed in shaded pools and streams in contrast to the sun loving *An. maculatus*. The main vectors in Sabah are *An. sundaicus* and *An. balabacensis*. Chloroquine resistance in Malaysia was reported since 1963. First-line of treatment is Fansidar (Sulfadoxine + Pyrimethamine) in Sabah, Chloroquine and Fansidar in Peninsular Malaysia and Chloroquine in Sarawak [1].

Malaria deaths have remained relatively stable over the 1992-2003 periods, within a range of 21 to 40 deaths annually. Reported malaria deaths decreased to 21 in 1999, but then increased to 35 in 2000, 38 in 2002 and the latest 21 cases in 2003. Incidence rates increased during the early 1990s, peaking at 2.99/1000 populations in 1994. Incidence rates have been significantly down since 1998 (0.63 in 1998, 0.56 in 2000 and 0.46 in 2002) [15]. Refer to table 1 below.

Majority of malaria cases in Malaysia (70%) were reported among the males and age more than five years old (90%). In 2003, most of the cases were reported in Sarawak (41%) followed by Sabah (28%) and Pahang (13%). Kuala Lumpur, Labuan, Melaka and Perlis reported the least number of cases, less than one percent each [15].

In Malaysia, organized anti malaria campaign began in 1901 through integrated parasitological and entomological surveillance systems, followed by the development of permanent anti-larval work. The Malaria Eradication Program (MEP) was started in Peninsular Malaysia in 1967. This program failed to achieve its desired objective but it has greatly reduced malaria cases in the country from about 500,000 cases annually before its introduction to about 30,000-60,000 cases in the 1970's. The World Health Organization in 1980 declared that it was no longer feasible to adopt the eradication strategy in most part of the world. This was mainly due to the difficulties faced by many countries in trying to meet the enormous resources required for the successful implementation of the strategy and the development of insecticide and drug resistance. Malaysia thus joined the rest of the world by coordinating malaria control with primary health care, but maintaining the main control activities which remained basically the same as those applied during the eradication period. This was replaced by the Malaria Control Program in 1980 and was extended to Sabah and

Sarawak in 1986. In 1995, the primary health-care approach to malaria control was adopted. In 1996, Sabah started its Five-Year Action Plan for malaria control. There was great success. In 1995, Sabah was responsible for 84.2% of malaria cases in Malaysia, but in 2003, this has reduced to merely 27.9%. Malaria in Malaysia will be more confined to rural population living in less accessible and hilly forested hinterland with inadequate transportation and communication facilities. More attention must be provided to reduce malaria in these areas. Long–term infrastructure development and socioeconomic improvement are needed in these areas [15 – 16].

Table 1: Malaria reported cases annually, malaria deaths and incidence rates /1000 population from 1990-2003. (Source: Ministry of Health, Malaysia, 2004 and WHO, 2002, 2005)

	Number of malaria cases (Annually)	Malaria deaths	Incidence rates/1000 population
1990	50,500		
1991	39,189		2.4
1992	36,853	24	1.9
1993	39,890	23	2.1
1994	58,985	28	2.99
1995	59,208	34	2.97
1996	52,060	40	2.45
1997	26,651	25	1.23
1998	13,491	26	0.63
1999	11,106	21	0.49
2000	12,705	35	0.56
2001	12,780	46	0.53
2002	11,019	38	0.46
2003	6,338	21	0.28

The Primary Malaria Control Strategy in Malaysia Include:

1. Early diagnosis and prompt treatment
2. Strengthening management and supervision
3. Capacity building through training
4. Improvement of local operations
5. Maintaining surveillance and monitor outbreaks
6. Selective and sustaining vector control through indoor residual spraying and use of Insecticide-Treated mosquito Nets (ITNs). The use of ITNs has contributed significantly in the reduction of malaria in this country.
7. Community involvement, integration with other public health activities and collaborative operations
8. Increase surveillance and screening of malaria among foreigners (25% of malaria in this country were among foreigners) [16].

Some factors contributing to the continued transmission of malaria are the development of drug resistant *Plasmodium falciparum*, changes in vector behavior, and ecological changes due to socio-economic reasons [4].

Recently a new source of malaria has been introduced into the country. These were from the immigrant workers (legal/illegal) and the large number of tourists coming into the country. The number of reported imported malaria cases has increased nationwide together with the increase incidence of drug resistance in South East Asia, which raised much concern among both health workers and clinicians [8, 10 – 11, 17 – 19].

History of Malaria in Malaysia

Malaria is a disease that has hampered economic development in the country (formerly known as Malaya). Malcolm Watson [20], one of the pioneer anti-malaria workers in Malaya recommended to the government, malaria control program of draining and filling the swampy areas with the resulting reduction in the incidence of malaria in Malaya. In 1899, the Institute of Medical Research (IMR) was started. IMR made very valuable contributions towards solving some of the problems connected with malaria and mosquitoes. Hamilton Wright, the first director of IMR published in 1901 studies on malaria and mosquito. Daniels, Stanton, Fletcher, Pratt and Leicester, all Directors of IMR also did research on malaria and mosquitoes and published their research work. The period from 1927 has been one of rapid progress in the field of malaria chemotherapy and drug prophylaxis owing to the discovery of synthetic drugs which could be used to supplement or replace quinine. Green, Wallace, Field and Niven have made valuable contributions to the subject of chemotherapy and chemoprophylaxis of malaria in Malaya [21].

Review of Malaria Research in Malaysia

1901 – 1948 (The Early Years)

- Research was carried out on **malarial fevers** of Malaya – the study of taxonomy and vector biology and on malarial control.
- In 1911, a system of subsoil drainage was devised for the control of *Anopheles maculatus*. This vector was later found to be the principle vector of malaria in most part of Peninsular Malaysia. The effort to conquer the mosquito vectors continued with the development of more permanent method after the First World War. In the states of Selangor, Perak and Penang, agitation ponds, automatic siphons and flushed gates were constructed to destroy *Anopheles* breeding sites [20].
- In 1948, Field Stain for the identification of malaria parasites in blood smears was developed by Dr Field, a director of IMR.

1963 – 1971

- Many papers were published on *P. falciparum* resistance to chloroquine in Malaysia [21 – 28].

- Research on vectors of malaria and effect of residual spraying with insecticides [29 - 32]
- Research on malaria in monkeys and other animals [33 - 41]
- Research on entomological aspects of the malaria eradication pilot project in Malaya [42 – 43]
- Research on *Anopheles maculatus*, a new vector and potential vector on mainland Malaya [44]
- Review research on Malaria at the Institute for Medical Research, Kuala Lumpur [45]
- Ecology of malaria in Malaya [46]
- Epidemiology of malaria [47 – 48]
- Jungle malaria in West Malaysia [49]
- *Plasmodium knowlesi* malaria in man in Malaysia. [50] Management of malaria in Malaysia. chloroquine-pyrimethamine treatment. [51 - 52]
- Malaria prophylaxis in Malaysia [53]
- Clinical and laboratory diagnosis of malaria [54]

1972-1980

- Chemotherapy of malaria. Falciparum malaria resistant to chloroquine suppression but sensitive to chloroquine treatment in West Malaysia [55 – 57]
- Malaria in animals [58 – 59]
- Clinical and laboratory diagnosis of malaria [60 -61]
- Research on malaria control [62].
- Prevalence of malaria among the Orang Asli [63]

1981-1990

- Prevalence study and epidemiology of malaria in Malaysia. Malaysia is a rapidly developing country where clearance of jungle for land development schemes and highways is necessary. Persons involved in these activities are continually exposed to malaria infection. *P. falciparum* resistance to chloroquine and mosquito resistance to insecticide were widespread. [3, 6, 63].
- Prevalence of malaria among the Orang Asli [64]
- Study on the chemotherapy of malaria in endemic areas in Malaysia [65]

1991-2000

- Prevalence of malaria among the Orang Asli [66]
- Immunological study of malaria in Malaysia [66]
- Risk behavior of malaria in Malaysia [67]
- Current status of malaria in Malaysia. Anti-malaria activities such as the use of impregnated bednets, the Primary Health Care approach and focal spraying activities remain the same. *Plasmodium falciparum* continues to be the predominant species [9, 68]
- Epidemiology and control of malaria in Malaysia [4, 97 -71]
- Malaria control, resistance and treatment program [72 – 73]
- Malaria: Prophylaxis and therapy [17, 74]

- Malaria, epidemiology, retrospective study in hospitals in Malaysia. The species of malaria reported were *Plasmodium falciparum*, *Plasmodium vivax* and *Plasmodium malariae*. The increase incidence of malaria among foreigners. Forest workers (loggers, rattan collectors and forest product gatherers) were the group most exposed to malaria, followed by plantation workers, aboriginal communities, army and police personnels [8, 10 – 12]
- Malaria and entomological studies. In Malaysia, there are 434 species of mosquitoes, representing 20 genera. Of these, 75 species are *Anopheles* and of these 75 species, only 9 have been reported as vectors: *An. maculatus, An. balabacensis, An. dirus, An. letifer, An. campestris, An. sundaicus, An. donaldi, An. leucosphyrus and An. flavirostris*. *Anopheles* was found to breed in paddy fields, fishponds, and rivers. Other less popular habitats were temporary pools, mountain streams, and spring wells [69, 75 – 82]
- Research on malaria diagnosis and detection. In malaria patients, glucose turnover was 20 % greater than patients with enteric fever. This increased glucose uptake in falciparum malaria may have implications for metabolic complications and their clinical management. The nested PCR assay is a sensitive technique for collecting accurate malaria epidemiologic data [83 - 87]

2001-2006

- Immunological study of malaria in Malaysia [88- 89]
- Malaria: Prophylaxis and therapy. Yapp and Yap reported that extracts of *Lansium domesticum* are a potential source for compounds with activity towards chloroquine-resistant strains of *P. falciparum* [90]
- Entomological study of malaria. Vector surveys in the Kinabatangan area of Sabah, found that *Plasmodium falciparum* was the predominant species and *Anopheles balabacensis* the primary vector. Malaria cases have dropped drastically over the years. The study showed that space application of larvicides/adulticides or a mixture of both is able to reduce the malaria vector population and the malaria transmission. Report of *Anopheles latens* as the vector of *P. knowlesi* among humans and monkeys in Sarawak, Malaysia [14, 91 – 93]
- Malaria , epidemiology, clinical features, retrospective study in hospitals in Malaysia. Prevalence and distribution of these parasites, the problems associated with parasitic infections, the control measures taken to deal with these parasites and implications for the future. The increasing importance of import malaria among foreigners [13, 94 – 97]
- Prevalence study of malaria among the Orang Asli in Malaysia [97 – 99]
- Malaria control [100]
- Research on malaria diagnosis. This study found the diagnostic utility of the Cell-Dyn 4000 hematology analyzer's depolarization analysis in determining the sensitivity and specificity in malaria diagnosis. This approach is useful where there is no clinical suspicion of malaria [101]
- Study has found that *P. knowlesi* infection was misdiagnosed microscopically as *P. malariae*. This necessitates the use of molecular methods for correct identification [102]

REFERENCES

[1] Palmer K. Combating Communicable Diseases, World Health Organization 2002. http://www.wpro.who.int/themes_focuses/theme 1/focus2/tlf2malaysia.asp

[2] Thomas V and Dissanaike AS. Malaria endemicity among Orang Asli (Malaysian aborigines) as determined by indirect fluorescent antibody tests. *Am J Trop Med Hyg* 1977 Jul; 26 (4): 602-6.

[3] Oothuman P. Status of malaria in Malaysia. *The Family Practitioner* 11 1988; (1): 81-3.

[4] Mak JW, Jegathesan M, Lim PK, Hakim SL, Rain AN Ambu S, Chong HK. Epidemiology and control of malaria in Malaysia. *Southeast Asian J Trop Med Public Health* 1992 Dec;23(4):572-7.

[5] Rahman WA, Che' Rus A and Ahmad AH. Malaria and *Anopheles* mosquitoes in Malaysia. *Southeast Asian J Trop Med Public Health* 1997 Sep;29(3):537-40.

[6] Ministry of Health (MOH). Vector-borne diseases annual report. Ministry of health Malaysia 2000: 19-33.

[7] Chuah SK. Report of 59 malaria cases and the treatment and management of complications seen at the District Hospital, Kuala Kangsar, Perak, over a two-year period, from July 1982-June 1984. *J of the Malaysian Society of Health* 1985;5(1):25-30.

[8] Sidhu PS and Ng SC. A retrospective study on malaria cases admitted to the University Hospital, Kuala Lumpur, 1984-1988. *Med J Malaysia* 1991 Jun;46(2):177-82.

[9] Lim ES. Current status of malaria in Malaysia. *Southeast Asian J Trop Med Public Health* 1992 Sep;23 Suppl 4:43-9.

[10] Moore CS, Cheong I. Audit of imported and domestic malaria cases at Kuala

[11] Lumpur Hospital.*Br J Clin Pract* 1995; 49(6): 304-7

[12] Jamaiah I, Anuar AK, Najib NARN and Zurainee MN. Imported Malaria: A Retrospective Study in University Hospital, Kuala Lumpur, a ten-year experience. *Med J Malaysia* 1998 Mar; 53(1): 6-9

[13] Rahman WA, Adanan C R and Abu Hassan A. A study on some aspects of the epidemiology of malaria in an endemic district in Northern Peninsular Malaysia near Thailand border. *Southeast Asian J Trop Med Public Health* 1998 Sep;28(3):599-605.

[14] Koh KH, Chew PH and Kiyu A. A retrospective study of malaria infections in an intensive care unit of a general hospital in Malaysia. *Singapore Med J* 2004 Jan;45(1):28-36.

[15] Vythilingam I, Chan ST, Shanmugratnam C, *et al.* The impact of development and malaria control activities on its vectors in the Kinabatangan area of Sabah, East Malaysia. *Acta Trop* 2005 Oct; 96(1) :24-30.

[16] WHO. http://www.rbm.who.int/wmr2005/profiles/malaysia.pdf

[17] Matusop A and Tham AH. Prevention and Control of malaria. A historical perspective with particular response to Malaysia. Vector Journal 2006, Volume 4, Vector Borne Disease Control Section, Ministry Of Health Malaysia.

[18] Leo YS, Chew SK, Allen DM and Monteiro EH. Malaria: Prophylaxis and therapy. *Singapore Med J* 1994;35:509-11.

[19] Jamaiah I, Rohela M, Nissapatorn V, Khoo BL, Khoo PS, Radhiyah M and Aisyah A. Malaria: a 10-year(1994-2003) retrospective study at University Malaya Medical

Center (UMMC), Kuala Lumpur, Malaysia. *Southeast Asian J Trop Med Public Health 2005* :60-3.

[20] Nissapatorn V, Lim YA, Jamaiah I *et al*. Parasitic infections in Malaysia: changing and challenges. *Southeast Asian J Trop Med Public Health 2005* :50-9.

[21] Watson M, Some pages from the history of the prevention of malaria. Glasgow 1935.

[22] Sandosham AA and Thomas V. Malariology (With special reference to Malaya). Singapore University Press, 1982:9-18.

[23] Mahoney LE Chloroquine-resistant falciparum malaria. *Lancet* 1968 Nov 23; 2(7578) :1139.

[24] McKelvey TP, Lundie AR, Vanreenen RM, *et al*. Chloroquine-resistant falciparum malaria among British service personnel in West Malaysia and Singapore. *Trans R Soc Trop Med Hyg* 1971; 65(3) :286-309.

[25] McKelvey TP, Lundie AR, Williams ED, *et al*. Chloroquine-resistant malaria in West Malaysia. *Br Med J* 1968 Dec 14; 4(5632) :703-4.

[26] Sandosham AA. Chloroquine-resistant falciparum malaria in Malaya. *Singapore Med J* 1963 Mar.:3-5.Sandosham AA, Eyles DE, Pull JH, *et al*. Chloroquine-resistant Falciparum malaria in a semi-immune indigenous population in North Malaya. *Med J Malaya* 1966 Dec; 21(2) :115-24.

[27] Contacos PG, Lunn JS, Coatney GR. Drug-resistant falciparum malaria from Cambodia and Malaya. *Trans R Soc Trop Med Hyg* 1963 Nov.:417-24.

[28] Montgomery R, Eyles DE. Chloroquine resistant falciparum malaria in Malaya. *Trans R Soc Trop Med Hyg* 1963 Nov.:409-16.

[29] Clyde DF, DuPont HL, Miller RM, *et al*. Prophylactic and sporontocidal treatment of chloroquine resistant Plasmodium falciparum from Malaya. *Trans R Soc Trop Med Hyg* 1970; 64(6) :834-8.

[30] Moorhouse DE, Chooi CK. Notes on the bionomics of *Anopheles campestris*, reid, and on its disappearance following house-spraying with residual insecticides. *Med J Malaysia* 1964 Mar.:184-92.

[31] Cheng FY Responses of *Anopheles balabacensis* to various patterns of DDT-spraying of shelters in Sabah, East Malaysia. *Bull World Health Organ* 1968; 38(3) :469-77.

[32] Moorhouse DE, Wharton RH Studies on Malayan vectors of malaria; methods of trapping, and observations on biting cycles. *J Med Entomol* 1965 Jan.:359-70.

[33] Wharton RH, Laing AB, Cheong WH. Studies on the distribution and transmission of malaria and filariasis among aborigines in Malaya. *Ann Trop Med Parasitol* 1963 Jun.:235-54.

[34] Das SK, Strauss JM, Chee CT *Plasmodium inui*-like infection producing a presumably fatal illness in a leaf monkey *Presbytis johnii*--a previously undescribed host. *Med J Malaya* 1966 Jun; 20(4) :323.

[35] Coatney GR The simian malarias: zoonoses, anthroponoses, or both? *Am J Trop Med Hyg* 1971 Nov; 20(6) :795-803.

[36] Dunn FL Blood parasites of Southeast Asian primitive primates. *J Parasitol* 1964 Apr.:214-6.

[37] Cheong WH, Omar AH *Anopheles maculatus*, a new vector of *Wuchereria bancrofti* in Malaysia (Pulau Aur) and a potential vector on mainland Malaya. *Med J Malaya* 1965 Sep; 20(1) :74-5.

[38] Cheong WH, Sandosham AA, Coombs GL, *et al.* New isolations of P. cynomologi and P. inui from A. b. balabacensis in Perlis. *Med J Malaya* 1965 Sep; 20(1) :52.

[39] Cheong WH, Omar HB, Warren M, *et al. Anopheles Balabacensis balabacensis* identified as a vector of monkey malaria in Malaya. *Med J Malaya* 1965 Sep; 20(1) :76.

[40] Cheong WH, Warren M, Omar AH, *et al. Anopheles Balabacensis balabacensis* identified as vector of simian malaria in Malaysia. *Science* 1965 Dec 3; 150(701) :1314-5. Cheong WH, Ben Omar AH, Warren M. The known vectors of simian malaria in Malaya today. *Med J Malaya* 1966 Jun; 20(4) :327-9.

[41] Chin W, Contacos PG, Coatney GR, *et al.* A naturally acquited quotidian-type malaria in man transferable to monkeys. *Science* 1965 Aug 20.:865.

[42] Collins WE, Skinner JC, Guinn EG, *et al.* Fluorescent antibody reactions against six species of simian malaria in monkeys from India and Malaysia. *J Parasitol* 1965 Feb.:81-4.

[43] Huehne WH, Ahmad MD, Seng LD, *et al.* A comprehensive account of the malaria eradication pilot project in Malaya. *Med J Malaya* 1966 Sep; 21(1) :3-25.

[44] Moorhouse DE Some entomological aspects of the malaria eradication pilot project in Malaya. *J Med Entomol* 1965 Jun; 2(2) :109-19.

[45] Cheong WH, Fredericks HJ, Omar AH, *et al.* The incrimination of *Anopheles maculatus* as the vector of human malaria at the Kelantan-Thai border. *Med J Malaya* 1968 Mar; 22(3) :245.

[46] Sandosham AA Recent researches on Malaria at the Institute for Medical Research, Kuala Lumpur. *Med J Malaya* 1967 Dec; 22(2) :145-60.

[47] Collins WE, Warren M, Skinner JC, *et al.* Studies on the relationship between fluorescent antibody response and ecology of malaria in Malaysia. *Bull World Health Organ* 1968; 39(3) :451-63.

[48] Yap LF, Ramachandran CP, Balasingam E A parasitological study of Pulau Pinang and Pulau Perhentian Kechil, off Trengganu, West Malaysia. I. Malaria and filariasis. *Med J Malaya* 1968 Dec; 23(2) :118-22.

[49] Sandosham AA Malaria in rural Malaya. *Med J Malaya* 1970 Mar; 24(3) :221-6.

[50] Warren M, Cheong WH, Fredericks HK, *et al.* Cycles of jungle malaria in West Malaysia. *Am J Trop Med Hyg* 1970 May; 19(3) :383-93.

[51] Fong YL, Cadigan FC, Coatney GR A presumptive case of naturally occurring *Plasmodium knowlesi* malaria in man in Malaysia. *Trans R Soc Trop Med Hyg* 1971; 65(6) :839-40.

[52] Huehne WH Barrier spraying at the Kelantan side of the Thai-Malaysia border. *J Trop Med Hyg* 1971 May; 74(5) :106-9.

[53] Huehne WH Experience with an insecticide-drug combination and observations on suppressive chloroquine-pyrimethamine treatment. *J Trop Med Hyg* 1971 May; 74(5) :110-6.

[54] O'Holohan DR, Hugoe-Matthews J Malaria suppression and prophylaxis on a Malaysian rubber estate:sulformethoxine-pyrimethamine single monthly dose vs chloroquine single weekly dose. *Southeast Asian J Trop Med Public Health* 1971 Jun; 2(2) :164-8.

[55] Saha N, Banerjee B Erythrocyte G-6-PD deficiency among Chinese and Malays of Singapore. *Trop Geogr Med* 1971 Jun; 23(2) :141-4.

[56] Andre RG, Cadigan FC, Fredericks HJ, *et al.* In vivo and in vitro studies of chloroquine-resistant malaria in West Malaysia. *Trans R Soc Trop Med Hyg* 1972; 66(4) :644-52. 56.

[57] Lewis AN, Dondero TJ, Ponnampalam JT Letter: Falciparum malaria resistant to chloroquine suppression but sensitive to chloroquine treatment in West Malaysia. *Trans R Soc Trop Med Hyg* 1973; 67(2) :310-2.

[58] Lewis AN, Ponnampalam JT . Suppression of malaria with monthly administration of combined sulphadoxine and pyrimethamine. *Ann Trop Med Parasitol* 1975 Mar; 69(1) :1-12.

[59] Killick-Kendrick R, Garnham PC, Cheong WH, *et al.* Exoerythrocytic schizonts of *Plasmodium silvaticum* of the orang-utan. *Southeast Asian J Trop Med Public Health* 1972 Sep; 3(3) :454.

[60] Collins WE, Contacos PG, Garnham PC, *et al. Plasmodium hylobati*: a malaria parasite of the gibbon. *J Parasitol* 1972 Feb; 58(1) :123-8. 60. Collins WE, Skinner JC The indirect fluorescent antibody test for malaria. *Am J Trop Med Hyg* 1972 Sep; 21(5) :690-5.

[61] O'Holohan DR, Hugoe-Matthews J Clinical and laboratory experiences of malaria in a Seremban medical practice during the two years: 1970-1971. *Med J Malaya* 1972 Sep; 27(1) :52-6.

[62] Bolton JM The control of malaria among the Orang Asli in West Malaysia. *Med J Malaya* 1972 Sep; 27(1) :10-9.

[63] Thomas V, Hock SK and Leng YP. Seroepidemiology of malaria: age-specific pattern of *Plasmodium falciparum* antibody, parasite and spleen rates among children in an endemic area in peninsular Malaysia. *Trop Doct* 1981 Oct; 11 (4): 149-54.

[64] Lambros C, Davis DR, Lewis GE, Antimalarial drug susceptibility of *Plasmodium falciparum* isolates from forest fringe dwelling aborigines (Orang Asli) of peninsular Malaysia. Am J Trop Med Hyg 1989 Jul; 41(1): 3-8.

[65] Navaratnam V, Musa M, Shamsuddin H, et al. Chemosuppression of malaria by the triple combination mefloquine/sulfadoxine/pyrimethamine: a field trial in an endemic area in Malaysia. *Trans R Soc Trop Med Hyg* 1989; 83 :755-59.

[66] Gordon DM, Davis DR, Lee M, Lambros C, Harrison BA, Samuel R, Campbell GH, Jegathesan M, Selvarajan K and lewis GE. Significance of circumsporozoite-specific antibody in the natural transmission of *Plasmodium falciparum*, *Plasmodium vivax* and *Plasmodium malariae* in an aboriginal (Orang Asli) population of central peninsular Malaysia. *Am J Trop Med Hyg* 1991 Jul; 45 (1): 49-56.

[67] Arasu GD. Risk behavior in malaria in Malaysia. *Southeast Asian J Trop Med Public Health* 1992;23 Suppl 1:51-6.

[68] Warrell DA. The 1996 Runme Shaw Memorial lecture: malaria—past, present and future. *Ann Acad Med Singapore* 1997 May;26(3):380-7.

[69] Chang MS, Doraisingam P, Hardin S, *et al.* Malaria and filariasis transmission in a village/forest setting in Baram District, Sarawak, Malaysia. *J Trop Med Hyg* 1995 Jun; 98(3) :382-6.

[70] Hii J, Alexander N, Chuan CK, *et al.* Lambdacyhalothrin impregnated bednets control malaria in Sabah, Malaysia. *Southeast Asian J Trop Med Public Health* 1995 Jun; 26(2) :371-4.

[71] Leake DW, Hii JL Observations of human behavior influencing the use of insecticide-impregnated bednets to control malaria in Sabah, Malaysia. *Asia Pac J Public Health* 1994; 7(2) :92-7.

[72] Lokman Hakim S, Sharifah Roohi SW, Zurkurnai Y, *et al. Plasmodium falciparum*: increased proportion of severe resistance (RII and RIII) to chloroquine and high rate of resistance to sulfadoxine-pyrimethamine in Peninsular Malaysia after two decades. *Trans R Soc Trop Med Hyg* 1996 May-Jun; 90(3) :294-7.

[73] Hii JL, Chee KC, Vun YS, *et al.* Sustainability of a successful malaria surveillance and treatment program in a Runggus community in Sabah, East Malaysia. *Southeast Asian J Trop Med Public Health* 1996 Sep; 27(3) :512-21.

[74] Mordi MN, Mansor SM, Navaratnam V, *et al.* Single dose pharmacokinetics of oral artemether in healthy Malaysian volunteers. *Br J Clin Pharmacol* 1997 Apr; 43(4) :363-5.

[75] Kittayapong P, Clark JM, Edman JD, *et al.* Survey of the *Anopheles maculatus* complex (Diptera: Culicidae) in peninsular Malaysia by analysis of cuticular lipids. *J Med Entomol* 1993 Nov; 30(6) :969-74.

[76] Rahman WA, Abu Hassan A, Adanan CR, *et al.* The prevalence of *Plasmodium falciparum* and *P. vivax* in relation to *Anopheles maculatus* densities in a Malaysian village. *Acta Trop* 1993 Dec; 55(4) :231-5.

[77] Rahman WA, Abu Hassan A, Adanan CR Seasonality of *Anopheles aconitus* mosquitoes, a secondary vector of malaria, in an endemic village near the Malaysia-Thailand border. *Acta Trop* 1993 Dec; 55(4) :263-5.

[78] Rahman WA, Abu Hassan A, Adanan CR, *et al.* A report of *Anopheles* (Diptera: Culicidae) attracted to cow bait in a malaria endemic village in Peninsular Malaysia near the Thailand border. *Southeast Asian J Trop Med Public Health* 1995 Jun; 26(2) :359-63.

[79] Vythilingam I, Foo LC, Chiang GL, *et al.* The impact of permethrin impregnated bednets on the malaria vector *Anopheles maculatus* (Diptera: Culicidae) in aboriginal villages of Pos Betau Pahang, Malaysia. *Southeast Asian J Trop Med Public Health* 1995 Jun; 26(2) :354-8.

[80] Chang MS, Hii J, Buttner P, Mansoor F. Changes in abundance and behaviour of vector mosquitoes induced by land use during the development of an oil palm plantation in Sarawak. *Trans R Soc Trop Med Hyg* 1997 Jul-Aug; 91(4) :834-8.

[81] Seng CM, Matusop A, Sen FK. Differences in *Anopheles* composition and malaria transmission in the village settlements and cultivated farming zone in Sarawak, Malaysia. *Southeast Asian J Trop Med Public Health 1999 Sep*; 30(3) :454-9.

[82] Yap HH, Chong NL, Lee CY, *et al.* Field-simulated residual efficacy of betacyfluthrin against *Anopheles sinensis* Wiedemann. *Southeast Asian J Trop Med Public Health* 1997 Mar; 28(1) :233-4.

[83] Kano S, Onda T, Matsumoto Y, *et al.* Serological evaluation of malaria patients in Thailand: antibody response against electrophoresed antigenic polypeptides of *Plasmodium falciparum*. *Southeast Asian J Trop Med Public Health* 1998 Jun; 29(2) :341-3.

[84] Khoo A, Furuta T, Abdullah NR, *et al.* Nested polymerase chain reaction for detection of *Plasmodium falciparum* infection in Malaysia. *Trans R Soc Trop Med Hyg* 1996 Jan-Feb; 90(1) :40-1.

[85] Singh B, Cox-Singh J, Miller AO, *et al.* Detection of malaria in Malaysia by nested polymerase chain reaction amplification of dried blood spots on filter papers. *Trans R Soc Trop Med Hyg* 1996 Sep-Oct; 90(5) :519-21.

[86] Singh B, Choo KE, Ibrahim J, *et al.* Non-radioisotopic glucose turnover in children with falciparum malaria and enteric fever. *Trans R Soc Trop Med Hyg* 1998 Sep-Oct; 92(5) :532-7.

[87] Singh B, Bobogare A, Cox-Singh J, *et al.* A genus- and species-specific nested polymerase chain reaction malaria detection assay for epidemiologic studies. *Am J Trop Med Hyg* 1999 Apr; 60(4) :687-92.

[88] Conway DJ, Machado RL, Singh B, *et al.* Extreme geographical fixation of variation in the *Plasmodium falciparum* gamete surface protein gene Pfs48/45 compared with microsatellite loci. *Mol Biochem Parasitol* 2001 Jul; 115(2) :145-56.

[89] Cox-Singh J, Zakaria R, Abdullah MS, *et al.* Short report: differences in dihydrofolate reductase but not dihydropteroate synthase alleles in *Plasmodium falciparum* isolates from geographically distinct areas in Malaysia. *Am J Trop Med Hyg* 2001 Jan-Feb; 64(1-2) :28-31.

[90] Yapp DT, Yap SY *Lansium domesticum*: skin and leaf extracts of this fruit tree interrupt the lifecycle of Plasmodium falciparum, and are active towards a chloroquine-resistant strain of the parasite (T9) in vitro. *J Ethnopharmacol* 2003 Mar; 85(1) :145-50.

[91] Hassan AA, Rahman WA, Rashid MZ, *et al.* Composition and biting activity of *Anopheles* (Diptera: Culicidae) attracted to human bait in a malaria endemic village in peninsular Malaysia near the Thailand border. *J Vector Ecol* 2001 Jun; 26(1) :70-5.

[92] Seleena P, Lee HL, Chooi KH, *et al.* Space spraying of bacterial and chemical insecticides against *Anopheles balabacensis* Baisas for the control of malaria in Sabah, East Malaysia. *Southeast Asian J Trop Med Public Health* 2004 Mar; 35(1) :68-78.

[93] Vythilingam I, Tan CH, Asmad M, *et al.* Natural transmission of *Plasmodium knowlesi* to humans by *Anopheles latens* in Sarawak, Malaysia. *Trans R Soc Trop Med Hyg* 2006 May 23.

[94] Abdullah MR, Smith DH, Macfarlane SJ, Omar J and Singh B. Malaria: re-establishing clinical features. Paper presented at 2nd ICPTM 2001 October 9-1.

[95] Nimir AR, Isa NH, Eugene CB, *et al.* Severity of Malaria cases reported in urban and rural hospitals in Malaysia. *Southeast Asian J Trop Med Public Health* 2006 Sep; 37(5) :831-7.

[96] Singh B, Cox-Singh J Parasites that cause problems in Malaysia: soil-transmitted helminths and malaria parasites. *Trends Parasitol* 2001 Dec; 17(12) :597-600.

[97] Jamaiah I, Rohela M, Nissapatorn V, Mohamad Azlan H, Nor Adli AR, Shahrul Rizan I, Anez A and Jasmin B.A retrospective prevalence of malaria in an aborigine hospital in Gombak, Selangor, Malaysia. *Southeast Asian J Trop Med Public Health* 2006; 37(suppl 3): 1-4.

[98] Mahdy MAK, Chan BTE, Noor Hayati MI, Sa'iah HA, Ismail MG and Jeffrey J. The distribution of malaria parasites among Orang Asli populations living in the interior areas of Pahang and Kelantan, Malaysia. *Trop Biomed* 2004; 21(1): 101-105.

[99] Norhayati M, Rohani AK, Hayati MI, *et al.* Clinical Features of Malaria in Orang Asli population in Pos Piah, Malaysia. *Med J Malaysia* 2001 Sep;56 (3): 271-4.

[100] Rohani A, Zamree I, Lim LH, *et al*. Comparative field evaluation of residual-sprayed deltamethrin WG and deltamethrin WP for the control of malaria in Pahang, Malaysia. *Southeast Asian J Trop Med Public Health* 2006 Nov; 37(6) :1139-48.

[101] Josephine FP, Nissapatorn V Malaria: the value of the automated depolarization analysis. *Southeast Asian J Trop Med Public Health* 2005.:68-72.

[102] Singh B, Kim Sung L, Matusop A, *et al*. A large focus of naturaly acquired *Plasmodium knowlesi* infections in human beings. *Lancet* 2004 Mar 27; 363(9414) :1017-24.

Chapter 17

BIONOMICS OF MALARIA VECTORS IN SOUTHEAST ASIA

Indra Vythilingam*

*Parasitology Unit, Institute for Medical Research, Jalan Pahang, 50588 Kuala Lumpur, Malaysia

ABSTRACT

Although malaria vectors have been studied for decades, it is important to update this information as the ecology and landscape is changing all the time. The main aim of this review is to explore the vectors of malaria in Southeast Asia comprising of Cambodia, Laos, Malaysia, Myanmar, Thailand and Vietnam.

INTRODUCTION

The main aim of this review is to explore the vectors of malaria in Southeast Asia comprising of Cambodia, Laos, Malaysia, Myanmar, Thailand and Vietnam. This topic has been reviewed extensively by Macdonald [1], Reid [2], Kondrachine [3], Chow [4], Pholsena [5]. This is not a detailed review of the malaria vectors in the region but to highlight the current vectors in the region and their role in malaria transmission.

During the last ten years valuable knowledge on the bionomics of malaria vectors has been obtained from Cambodia, Laos, Myanmar and Vietnam. However, the bionomics of malaria vectors has been extensively studied in Malaysia and Thailand [2, 6] over the years. A detailed review of *An. dirus* has been published by Obsomer *et al* [7]. Due to extensive vector control measures and development many of the malaria vectors have disappeared from their original localities in Malaysia. However, in Thailand the vectors are still predominant in many areas.

Table 1. Malaria Vector Species in Southeast Asia

Country	Primary	Secondary	Suspected
Cambodia	*An. dirus, An. minimus*	*An. sundaicus*	*An. maculatus*
Laos	*An. dirus, An. minimus*	*An. jeyporensis*	*An. nivipes, An. maculatus*
Malaysia	*An. maculatus, An. balabacensis, An. latens*	*An. sundaicus An. donaldi*	
Myanmar	*An. dirus, An. minimus*	*An. culicifacies An. sinensis, An. jeyporensis*	*An. aconitus, An. annularis, An. maculatus, An. philippinensis, An. sundaicus*
Thailand	*An. dirus, An. minimus*	*An. maculatus, An. sundaicus*	*An. aconitus*
Vietnam	*An. dirus, An. minimus*	*An. sundaicus, An. subpictus*	*An. maculatus*

The predominant vectors in this region are shown in Table 1. This is still not a complete picture. In many areas of Lao PDR the vectors remain unknown. There have also been changes to the names of some of these vectors. Only about 30-40 species are known to transmit malaria and of these Southeast Asia has one of the most numbers of malaria vector species. It is important to know the biology, ecology and behaviour of vectors in order to determine its role in malaria transmission and to institute appropriate control measures against the vectors. Although malaria vectors have been studied for decades, it is important to update this information as the ecology and landscape is changing all the time.

Distribution

Anopheline vectors differ in different areas according to the nature of the terrain and its vegetation. Thus a country can be broadly classified into three main zones – the brackish water zone, the coastal plain and the hilly mountainous and forested region. Within these regions it can be further subdivided based on whether the land has been cleared of jungle and cultivated. However, there is no hard and fast rule between these zones. They can extend 500km or more into neighbouring areas.

The brackish water zone can again be divided into two: along the coast and in untouched mangrove swamp where no vector species of Anophelines breed. Where the mangrove has been cleared and the tidal waters allowed to come in contact with the exposed collections of fresh water, *An. sundaicus* can breed. This is a good vector of malaria. *An. sundaicus* prefers full exposure to sunlight. It will breed in water in varying salinity from almost that of sea water to water which is almost fresh. Most intense breeding occurs between 10-20% salinity. Its favourite breeding places are those with stagnant water exposed to sunlight, such as small open pools, large shallow wells and earth drains [8]. *An. sundaicus* has also been found breeding inland, presumably in fresh water, in Sarawak, Malaysia [9]. Molecular studies carried out has provided evidence that *An. sundaicus* ss exist on Borneo Island while in Cambodia, peninsular Malaysia, Thailand and Vietnam this species has now been given a new name *An. epiroticus* [10].

The hills and mountains intersected by numerous valleys form the backbone of the peninsula Malaysia which is for the greater part clothed in heavy tropical jungle. In virgin hill jungle it is possible to find members of the *An. lecucosphyrus* species group. However, when the cover of the jungle is removed from hilly areas, *An. maculatus*, our most important vector breeds. *Anopheles maculatus* breeds in slow flowing streams exposed to sunlight. It occurs from foothills to the tops of mountains at 5,000 feet above sea level. It is found in great numbers where there has been recent soil disturbance e.g. felling of trees and clearing [2]. *Anopheles maculatus* is an important vector in P. Malaysia and Southern Thailand. Although it has been found in large numbers in Laos [11], Cambodia and Vietnam [12] it is not a vector in these countries.

In Sabah (East Malaysia) about 80% of the country is hilly and forested. The country contains central mountain ranges from four to six thousand feet in height. The mountainous terrains are ideal for the breeding of the forest mosquito *An. balabacensis*. The most typical breeding places are formed by pools and seepages in deep shade in the jungle, where water is frequently replenished by rain. Animal foot prints in the jungle serve as good breeding sites.

In the coastal regions of Sabah *An. sundaicus* plays a role as vector, while *An. flavirostris* was found to be a vector in coastal parts of Banggi Island, Pitas and Semporna districts[13]. In the coastal region of Sarawak *An. sundaicus* has been found breeding in brackish water and it has also been found breeding inland in fresh water [14]. *An. donaldi* has also been found breeding in forest areas of Sabah and Sarawak and has been incriminated as a vector of malaria [15 – 16]. *An. donaldi* breeds in shady places on the edge of forest, mainly in hilly areas not far from swamp forest [8].

An. latens (previuoaly known as *An. lecucosphyrus,* [17]) is found in forested areas of Sarawak. It breeds in clear seepage pools besides streams in the jungle and in swampy patches [18].

Anopheles dirus is the main vector of malaria in Thailand, Vietnam, Cambodia, Laos and Myanmar [11 - 12, 16, 19 – 21]. *Anopheles dirus* is mainly a vector in the forested region of these countries. *Anopheles drius* is a species complex and in Thailand 5 species of the complex has been found [6]. Larvae *of An. dirus* typically breeds in small, often temporary, shaded pools of water in hilly regions of tropical, evergreen rainforest

An. minimus which is also a species complex [22] breeds mostly in slow moving waters such as streams, seepages and rivers with grassy edges [4]. With DDT spraying *An. minimus* was almost wiped out. It is a still an important vector in parts of Thailand and Vietnam [12, 23]. Although it was suspected to be a vector in Lao PDR studies in the Southern province of Lao PDR showed otherwise [11 - 12, 21, 24].

An. jeyporensis has been incriminated as a vector in Lao PDR [11] and in Vietnam in Di-Linh [4]. It occurs mainly in the hilly areas. The breeding sites are similar to those of *An. minimus*.

Larval Biology

Eggs of *Anopheles* mosquitoes are boat shaped and have lateral floats. The eggs are laid in water and will not survive desiccation. The larvae comprise of 4 instars of which the first and 2nd are very small and the hairs not very well defined. In *Anopheles* larvae the siphon is absent but palmate hairs are present. The larvae are surface feeders. The 4th instar larva moults to form the pupa.

Table 2. Behaviour of Anopheles Vectors Observed in Various Countries In Southeast Asia

Species	Country	Trophic preference	Resting preference	Biting preference	Source
An. balabacensis	Sabah (East Malaysia	Exophagic	Exophilic	Antropophgaic	Hii *et al.* 1988
An. dirus	Thailand	Exophagic	Exophilic	Antropophgaic	Baimai *et al.* 1988
An. dirus	Myanmar	Exophagic	Exophilic	Antropophagic/ Zoophagic	Aung *et al.* 1999
An. dirus	Myanmar		Exophilic	Antropophagic	Oo e*t al.* 2003
An. dirus	Cambodia	Endophagic	Exophilic	Antropophagic	Trung *et al.* 2005
An. dirus	Laos	Endophagic		Antropophagic	Vythilingam *et* al. 2005
An. dirus	Laos	Endophagic		Antropophagic	Toma *et al* 2002
An. dirus	Vietnam	Endophagic	Exophilic	Antropophagic	Trung *et al* 2005
An.jeyporensis	Laos	Endophagic		Antropophagic	Vythilingam *et al* 2003
An. latens	Sarawak (E Malaysia	Endophagic	Exophilic	Antropophagic	Colless 1965
An. latens	Sarawak (E Malaysia	Exophagic		Antropophagic/ Zoophagic	Vythilingam *et al* 2006
An. maculatus	Malaysia	Exophagic	Exophilic	Zoophagic/Antropophagic	Sandosham and Thomas 1982, Wharton 1953
An. maculatus	Malaysia	Exophagic		Antropophagic	Vythilingam *et al* 1995
An. maculatus	Laos	Exophagic	Exophilic		Vythilingam *et al* 2003
An. maculatus	Thailand	Exophagic	Exophilic	Zoophagic	Upatham *et al* 1988
An. maculatus	Vietnam	Exophagic	Exophilic	Zoophagic	Trung *et al* 2005
An. minimus A	Cambodia	Endophagic	Exophilic	Zoophagic	Trung *et al* 2005
An. minimus	Laos	Exophagic	Exophilic		Vythilingam *et al* 2003
An. minimus	Laos	Exophagic/Endophagic	Exophiliy	Antropophagic/ zoophagic	Toma et al 2002; Trung *et al* 2005
An. minimus	Thailand	Exophagic	Exophilic	Zoophagic	Ratanatham et al 1988
An. minimus	Vietnam	Endophagic	Endophilic	Antropophagic	Trung et al 2005
An. sundaicus	Malaysia	Endophagic	Endophilic		Sandosham & Thomas, 1982
An. sundaicus	Vietnam	Endophagic	Exophilic	Antropophagic	Trung *et al* 2005

Host Preference

An. maculatus bites cattle more than man [2, 25 – 26]. The preference of cattle to man is 2:1 [25]. Studies by Wharton [26] showed that *An. maculatus* was also attracted to both goats and dogs and to dogs more so than man. *An. balabacensis* prefers to bite man more than water buffalo, the ratio being 1.8:1 [13]. *An. latens* is anthropophilic; 78.8% fed on humans while the rest fed on dogs, pigs and fowls [27]. *An. latens* is also attracted to non human primates. The human: monkey biting ratio was 1:1.12 and bites monkey more at canopy than at ground [28]. In recent studies in Cambodia, Laos and Vietnam *An. dirus* showed extremely high preference for humans [29]. *Annopheles minimus* A was more anthropophilic than *An. minimus* C [29]. *An. sundaicus* is also highly anthropophilic. The behaviour of these mosquitoes from the different countries is shown in Table 2.

Resting Places

In Malaysia *Anopheles* mosquitoes in general do not remain indoors long after feeding with the exception of *An. Campestris* [8]. *An. maculatus* rests mostly on upper parts of walls of houses and on grass stems and bushes around cattle sheds at night [8, 26]. *An. maculatus* rests on outside of the house before entering [30] and attacks on entering houses and rest on wall after feeding [30 -31]. *An. balabacensis* also rests indoors after feeding and exits the same night or early morning [32]. *An. latens* rests on the walls before and after feeding and is usually found low down on the walls [33]. These mosquitoes are also known to rest on under surface of leaves before coming to feed. *An. dirus* is known to rest on the walls of wells in Myanmar [34]. *An. minimus* is considered a domestic species and thus found resting mainly indoors. They are found resting inside and behind mosquito nets, on clothes, underneath beds. Most found in the lower part of the walls [4]. *An. sundaicus* is also known to rest indoors before and after feeding. In Cambodia large numbers were found indoors in the daytime [4]. Like *An. minimus*, *An. jeyporensis* is also a domestic mosquito found resting indoors. Can also be found resting in cattle sheds [4].

Biting Activity

The biting activity of *An. maculatus* starts as early as 1930 hours and the peak occurs between 2230 -2330 and 0230 hours [35]. *An. balabacensis* bites more outdoors than indoors [36]. The peak biting time for *An. balabacensis* was between 1900 and 2000 hours but continued throughout the night outdoors. The peak biting indoors was between 2200 and 2300 hours [16]. *An. latens* bites humans from 1800 hours and peaks at midnight [28]. *Anopheles dirus* starts to bite as early as 1900 hours but the peak is around 2200 hours and continues to bite throughout the night until 0600 hours [6, 11, 29]. *An. jeyporensis* showed a steady increase around 2200 hours and declined steadily thereafter [11]. *An. sundaicus* exhibits a peak biting activity from 2000 until 0300 hours [37].

Gonotrophic Cycle

The duration of gonotrophic cycle of *An. balabacensis* in the field as determined by mark release recapture experiments was found to be 2-3 days [38], while that of *An. maculatus* was found to be 2.3 days [39 – 40]. Most of the species have a gonotrophic cycle of about 3 days.

Survivorship

The survivorship of *An. balabacensis* was high in Sabah ranging between 0.719 to 0.78 [13]. *An. maculatus* also had a similar survivorship of 0.71 to 0.761 [39] and 0.69-0.71 [40]. *An. dirus* and *An. latens* also have a high survivorship with values being more than 0.8 [11, 41 – 42].

Table 3. Sporozoite Rates Obtained From Various Species of *Anopheles* in Southeast Asia

Species	Country	Year	Sporozoite Rate %	Source
An. balabacensis	Sabah East Malaysia	1984	1.15-6.38	Hii *et al* 1988
An. dirus	Thailand	1984-1985	2-1.6	Upatham *et al* 1988
An. dirus	Thailand	1983-1985	0.4-4.1	Rosenberg *et al* 1990
An. dirus	Thailand	1983-1987	0.4-0.7	Gingrich *et al* 1990
An. dirus A	Laos	2000	0.55-0.81	Vythilingam *et al* 2003
An. dirus A	Laos	2002-2004	0.17-2.69	Vythilingam *et al* 2005
An. dirus A	Cambodia	1999	10.7	Trung *et al* 2004
An. dirus	Vietnam	1998-2000	1.1-1.2	Trung *et al* 2004
An. dirus	Myanmar	1998-2000	0.4-2.4	Oo *et al* 2003
An. jeyporensis	Laos	2000	2.5-4.5	Vythilingam *et al* 2003
An. jeyporensis	Vietnam		0.83	Chow 1970
An. latens	Sarawak East Malaysia	2005	1.18	Vythilingam *et al* 2006
An. latens	Sarawak East Malaysia	1994	0-0.42	Chang *et al* 1999
An. maculatus	Malaysia	1990-1992	0.02-1.24	Vythilingam et al 1995
An. maculatus	Malaysia	1960s	10-15	Sandosham & Thomas 1982
An. maculatus	Thailand	1984-1985	0	Upatham *et al* 1998
An. minimus	Thailand	1983-1985	0.5	Gingrich *et al* 1990
An. minimus A	Vietnam	1998-2000	2.8	Trung *et al* 2004
An. minimus	Cambodia	1999	1.4	Trung *et al* 2004
An. minimus	Laos	1956-1957	1.4	Chow 1970
An. sundaicus	Vietnam	1999-2000	0	Trung et al 2004
An. sundaicus	Malaysia		0.4	Sandosham & Thomas 1982

Vector Parasite Relationship

In order to be a good vector the *Anopheles* mosquitoes must be able to develop sporozoites. The presence of sporozoites indicates it is an efficient vector. Most of the species described above have been positive for sporozoites as shown in Table 3. In Thailand, *An. dirus* which used to be a forest species has now adapted to fruit orchards and plantations [41, 43]. It is important for species to live long enough and to develop the parasite to the infective stage before it can be considered as a good vector.

Vector control Indoor residual house spraying with DDT has been the main tool for malaria vector control for decades. Most of these countries had spraying programmes in an organized way at some point in time [44]. In 1990s the switch was made to insecticide treated bednets. Studies carried out in a malaria endemic area in Pos Betau, Pahang, Malaysia showed that with the use of permethrin treated bednets *An. maculatus* density and sporozoite rates decreased [35] compared to the area using placebo nets. In early years permethrin was the insecticide of choice for treating bednets and most countries using this additional tool reported lower incidence of cases [44]. However, countries should monitor the vector situation all the time since it has been shown that the behaviour of the vectors has changed over time [29]. It is a complex situation and one has to be vigilant especially when cases have been reduced to low levels. With rapid travel cases can be brought into the country at any time and epidemics can take place if proper control strategies are not in place. Thus, it is important to study the bionomics of vectors at least every 7-10 years.

REFERENCES

[1] Macdonald G. *The epidemiology and control of malaria.* London: Oxford University press, 1957.

[2] Reid JA. Anopheline mosquitoes of Malaya and Borneo. *Studies Institute for Medical Research Mala*ysia 1968; 31: 520.

[3] Kondrachine AV. Malaria in Southeast Asia. *Southeast Asian Journal of Tropical Medicine and Public Health* 1986; 17: 642-655.

[4] Chow CY. Bionomics of malaria vectors in the Western Pacific region. *Southeast Asian Journal of Tropical Medicine and Public Health* 1970; 1: 40-57.

[5] Pholsena K. The malaria situation and antimalaria program in Laos. *Southeast Asian Journal Tropical Medicine and Public Health* 1992; 23: 39-42.

[6] Baimai V, Harbach RE, Kijchalao U. Cytogenetic evidence for two species within the current concept of the malaria vector Anopheles leucosphyrus in Southeast Asia. *Journal of American Mosquito Control Association* 1988; 4: 44-50.

[7] Obsomer V, Defourny P, Coosemans M. The Aopheles dirus complex spatial distribution and environmental drivers. *Malaria Journal* 2007; 6: 6-26.

[8] Sandosham, AA. and Thomas, V. Malariology with special reference to Malaya. Singapore University Press. 1982: 382.

[9] Linton YM, Harbach RE, Chang MS, Anthony TG, Asmad M. Morphological and molecular identity of Anopheles (Cellia) sundaicus (Diptera: Culicidae), the

nominotypical member of a malaria vector species complex in Southeast Asia. *Systematic Entomology* 2001; 26: 357-366.

[10] Linton YM, Dusfour I, Howard TM, Ruiz LF, Nguyen DM, Trung HD, Sochanta T, Coosemans M, Harbach RE. Anopheles (Cellia) epiroticus (Diptera: Culicidae), a new malaria vector species in the Southeast Asian Sundaicus complex. *Bulletin of Entomological Research* 2005; 95: 329-339.

[11] Vythilingam I, Phetsouvanh R, Keokenchanh K, Yengmala V, Vanisaveth A, Phompida S, akim SL. The prevalence of Anopheles (Diptera: Culicidae) mosquitoes in Sekong Province, Lao PDR in relation to malaria transmission. *Tropical Medicine and International Health* 2003; 8: 525-535.

[12] Trung HD, Van Bortel W, Sochantha T, Keokenchanh K, Quang NT, Cong LD, Coosemans M. Malaria transmission and major malaria vectors in different geographical areas of Southeast Asia. *Tropical Medicine and International Health.* 2004; 9: 230-237

[13] Hii JLK, Vun YS. A study of the dispersal, survival and adult population estimates of the malaria, Anopheles balabacensis (baisas (Diptera: Culicidae) in Sabah Malaysia. *Tropical Biomedicine*. 1985; 2: 121-131.

[14] Chang MS, Linton YM, Harbach RE. The Anopheles sundaicus species complex – a preliminary study of larval ecology from two sites in Sarawak, Malaysia. Mekong *Malaria Forum* 2001; 8: 91-95.

[15] Chang MS, Hii J, Buttner P, Mansoor F. Changes in abundance and behaviour of vector mosquitoes induced by land use during development of an oil palm plantation in Sarawak. *Transactions of the Royal Society of Tropical Medicine and Hygiene* 1997; 91: 382-386.

[16] Vythilingam I, Sidavong B, Chan ST, Phonemixy T, Vanisaveth V, Sisoulad P, Phetsouvanh R, Lokman Hakim S, Phompida S. Epidemiology of malaria in Attapeu province Lao PDR in relation to entomological parameters. *Transactions of Royal Society of Tropical Medicine and Hygiene* 2005; 99: 833-839.

[17] Sallum MAM., Peyton EL, Wilkerson RC. Six new species of the Anopheles leucosphyrus group, reinterpretation of An. elegans and vector implications. *Medical and Veterinary Entomology* 2005; 19: 158-199.

[18] Colless DH. The Anopheles leucosphyrus group. *Transactions Royal Entomological Society London*. 1956; 108: 37-116.

[19] Baimai V, Kijchalao U, Sawadwongporn P, Green CA. Geographic distribution and biting behaviour of four species of the Anopheles dirus complex (Diptera: Culicidae) in Thailand. *Southeast Asian Journal of Tropical Medicine and Public Health* 1988; 19: 151-161.

[20] Paing MAA, Sebastain Lin T. Anopheline mosquitoes of Myanmar 1. Anopheles (Cellia) dirus Peyton and Harrison, 1979. *Myanmar Health Science Research Journal* 1989; 1: 122-129.

[21] Toma T, Miyagi I, Okazawa T, Kobayashi J, Saita S, Tuzuki A, Keomanila H, Nambanya A, Phompida S, Uza M, Takakura M. Entomological surveys of malaria in Khammouane province, Lao PDR, in 1999 and 2000. *Southeast Asian Journal Tropical Medicine and Public Health*. 2002; 33: 532-546.

[22] Van Bortel W, Trung HD, Manh ND, Roelants P, Verle P, Coosemans M. Identification of two species within the Anopheles minimus complex in northern Vietnam and their behavioural divergences. *Tropical Medicine International Health* 1999; 57-265.

[23] Ratanatham S, Upatham ES, Prasittisuk C, Rojanasunan W, Theeraslip N, Tremongkol A, Viyanant V. Bionomics of Anopheles minimus and its role in malaria transmission in Thailand. *Southeast Asian Journal Tropical Medicine and Public Health* 1988; 19: 283-289.

[24] Kobayashi J, Somboon P, Keomanila H, Inthavongsa S, Nambanya S, Inthakone S, Sato Y, Miyagi I. Malaria prevalence and brief entomological survey in a village surrounded by rice fields in Khammouan province, Lao PDR. *Tropical Medicine and International Health* 2000; 5: 17-21.

[25] Loong KP, Chiang GL, Yap HH. Field studies of the bionomics of Anopheles maculatus and its role in malaria transmission in Malaysia. *Southeast Asian Journal Tropical Medicine and Public Health* 1988; 19: 724.

[26] Wharton RH. The habits of adult mosquitoes in Malaya. I. Observations on Anophelines in window trap huts and at cattle-sheds. *Annals of Tropical Medicine and Parasitology* 1951; 45: 141-154.

[27] Colbourne MJ, Huehne WH, Lachance FS. TheSarawak anti-malaria project. *Sarawuk Museum Journal.* 1999; 9: 215 – 248.

[28] Vythilingam I, Tan CH, Asmad M, Chan ST, Lee KS, Singh B. Natural transmission of Plasmodium knowlesi to humans by Anopheles latens in Sarawak, Malaysia. *Transactions of Royal Society of Tropical Medicine and Hygiene* 2006; 10: 1087-1088.

[29] Trung HD, Van Bortel W, Sochantha T, Keokenchanh K, Oliver J, Briet T, Coosemans M. Behavioural heterogeneity of Anopheles species in ecologically different localities in Southeast Asia: a challenge for vector control. *Tropical Medicine and International Health* 2005; 10: 251-262.

[30] Moorhouse DE. Some entomological aspects of the malaria eradication pilot project in Malaya. *Journal of Medical Entomology* 1965; 2: 359-270.31.

[31] Reid JA, Wharton RH. Trials of residual insecticides in window-trap huts against Malayan mosquitoes. *Bulletin of Entomological Research* 1956; 47: 433-468.

[32] Hii JLK. Anopheles malaria vectors in Malaysia with reference to Sabah. In Hariansuta, C. Reynolds, DC (Eds) Problems of malaria in SEAMIC Countries. *Southeast Asian Medical Information Centre*: Tokyo, 1985; 71-81.

[33] Colless DH Observations on Anopheline mosquitoes of the Akah river, 4th division of Sarawak. *Bulletin Entomological Research* 1965; 47: 115-123.

[34] Oo TT, Storch V, Becker N. Anopheles dirus and its role in malaria transmission in Myanmar. *Journal of Vector Ecology*. 2003; 28: 175-183.

[35] Vythilingam I, Foo LC, Chiang GL, Chan ST, Eng KL, Mahadevan S, Mak JW, Inder Singh K. The impact of permethrin impregnated bednets on the malaria vector Anopheles maculatus (Diptera: Culicidae) in Aboriginal villages of Pos Betau, Pahang, Malaysia. *Southeast Asian Journal Tropical Medicine and Public Health.* 1995; 32; 4-358.

[36] Hii JLK, Kan S, Vun YS, Chin KF, Tambakau S, Chan MKC, Lye MS, Mak JW, Cochrane H. Transmission dynamics and estimates of malaria vectorial capacity for Anopheles balabacensis and An. flavirostris (Diptera:Culicidae) on Banggi islands, Sabah, Malaysia. *Annals of Parasitology and Tropical Medicine*. 1988; 82: 91-101.

Index

A

D

E

F

G

H

I

J

K

L

M

N

O

P

Q

R

S

T

U

V

W

Y

Z